"Game-changer ... *Breath:* transformative guide that empowers ... lifestyle through the power of breath. Through insightful wisdom ... practical guidance, Dr. Jeannie May highlights the profound impact of our breath on regulating our nervous system, fostering inner calm, and tapping into our inherent resilience and wisdom. This thought-provoking and inspiring book beautifully articulates the profound impact of breath work on our overall well-being. It is an invaluable resource for those looking to cultivate a deeper connection with themselves, find inner peace, and embrace a more conscious and fulfilling way of living.

-Deborah Giles, Founder & CEO
Center for Technology

"So informative and mind-bending! I've known Dr. Jeannie May for more than six years, and she is a prolific author and scholar of growth, development, and wellness in mind and body. Her compassion as a physician shines through in her newest book, *Breath: The Remote Control to Inner Calm.* In this work, she explores the human body with a depth of detail only a physician could provide. She explains the A-Z of breathing, emphasizing its importance and significance in promoting healing, calm, and stress relief. I have attended her Breathwork sessions, and no matter how much inner work I've done to overcome life's obstacles, each session she guides uncovers deeply seeded issues that I wasn't aware needed to be released. This practice brings about a profound sense of relief, gratitude, and freedom. I highly recommend this book. It reflects Dr. May's heart, soul, and dedication to helping others achieve greater freedom and transformation in their lives."

-Tammy De Mizra

"Dr. Jeannie May's Breathwork book and journeys have opened up new realms of healing and transformation for me and many others. Her writing style is potent, relatable, accessible, and playful while grounded in firm science and technical know-how. Her dedication to helping us individually and collectively heal the stress epidemic we're living in is noble and inspiring, particularly as the solution is simple, practical, and universally available: the breath. This is a must read for anyone who wants to claim their inner peace, health, and longevity."

-Caitlin Elise Nisos

The Breathwork Experience With Dr. Jeannie May

"This experience was life-changing. Things from my past processed as energy moved through my body, and I was feeling so good for days afterwards. Dr. Jeannie May is made for this. Her voice is so soothing and helped me to relax and get into the space so much faster. This work is amazing."

-Sandie Cuchinelli

"Dr. Jeannie's Breathwork sessions have been exceptionally helpful to my well being. I released long-held animosities that have kept me from freeing myself from past traumas. Highly recommend."

-Ann Raines

"My Breathwork sessions with Dr. Jeannie May are so powerful and loving. Each one is different every time with my last session resulting in a huge healing. Dr. May was born to do this work and is helping so many people in this healing journey."

-Maria Alicia Lopez

"At different times I could feel the hurting and then the letting go in my body, especially in my thoracic area and around my spine which are always very tight and sore. Then I felt my whole ribcage expand deeper which was a new sensation. I have not breathed that deeply in my lungs for a long time. I was so much more relaxed by the end. I felt honored and not pushed—Dr. Jeannie May is very good at this."

-RA

"Anytime I can connect with my body, I love it. At one point it felt like I was feeling colors – if that makes any sense. Darker colors were becoming lighter. I have chronic pain in the right side of my torso and right arm, and I could feel something heavy let go as I felt a connection between the two. I am very appreciative for the experience."

-Deb Knapp

"I felt like a new person. It really helped with my depression and anxiety. I was relaxed for days."

-Dell Walker

"Breathwork is a very therapeutic experience. It felt like very good energy as I gained clarity that I am on the right path to making myself a better life by doing the work to heal. I have done Breathwork in group settings, and I really enjoyed my session with Dr. Jeannie May in the comfort of my own room by myself. When I was in the group setting, I kept getting distracted by the other people wondering if I was doing it wrong and comparing myself to them. I tell everyone about this – if they want a quicker way to deal with their past traumas and to speed up their healing, this is the way to do it. I am very appreciative for this work."

-SK

"Breathwork with Dr. Jeannie May is a must! Her voice is soothing, her music choices are thoughtful and her ability to create a welcoming environment is undeniable! Each session is its own journey and a worthwhile investment in personal development."

-Auti S

"I was skeptical about Breathwork at first, but Dr. Jeannie May's compassionate guidance and expertise made me a believer. I've never felt more grounded and centered."

-John Raines

"Dr. Jeannie May helped me explore my body's pain while giving myself permission to feel emotions tied to that pain. I felt heard and seen."

-Jo Justian

"I recently did a Breathwork session with Dr. Jeannie May, TheBreathMD. During my session, I felt energy move through my body. I released so much emotion that had not been fully processed, and I was shocked at how transformative her process was for me. The week following my session, I had such ease, less weight, and a clearer sense of power that I was able to work more freely and felt a newer state of calm. I had no idea just how much frenetic energy I was walking around with before going through such a release! I highly recommend this to any individual or leader looking to progress their life from where they are to where they want to be."

-Janet Alexander

"This was a very healing experience. It was like I was breathing in love and light and dispelling the darkness and shadows for the betterment of my body and soul."

-Philip Raines

"It's quite fitting that Dr. Jeannie May be the one who facilitates Breathwork sessions, because only a medical doctor, with her knowledge of the human body, could lead a group of people to such powerful healing! I can tell you that you can heal both the mind and the body just by taking deep breaths. After a Breathwork session, I feel an amazing sense of peace and clarity, my mind no longer races, and the built up tension in my body significantly decreases. The loving and encouraging messages you hear from Dr. May, during the sessions, along with the mental state the deep breathing puts you in, causes you to slowly change the negative, self-hating belief systems many of us have buried in our subconscious minds. You start to see yourself from a more loving and forgiving place, which causes you to begin seeing everything else in that same light. It's transformational! Dr. May's Breathwork sessions are going to completely revolutionize medicine, and I hope you give yourself a chance to experience healing as well!"

-James Hayes

" There is one way of breathing that is shameful and restricted. Then, there's another way: A breath of love that takes you to infinity." -Rumi

Breath
The Remote Control to Inner Calm

Jeannie May M.D.

Breath
The Remote Control to Inner Calm

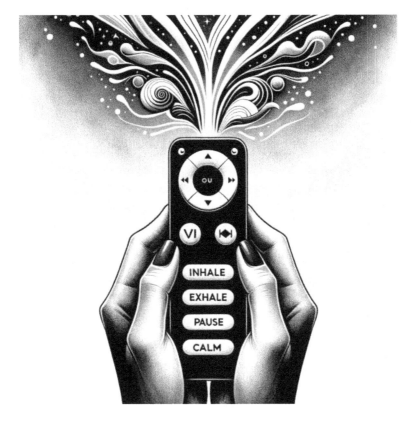

Jeannie May, M.D.
TheBreathMD

Breath: The Remote Control to Inner Calm
JLM Publishing Trust formerly JACC Publishing
Nashville, TN

ISBN: 978-0-9991861-1-4

May MD, Jeannie.
Breath: The Remote Control to Inner Calm / Jeannie May MD
-1st Edition.

Printed in the United States.

www.TheBreathMD.com

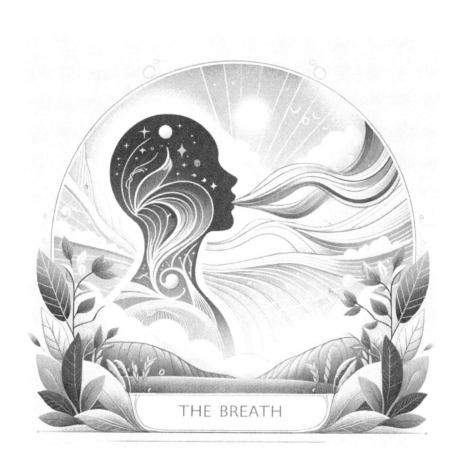

THE BREATH

**When you own your breath,
Nobody can steal your peace.**

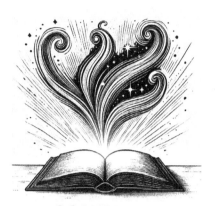

CONTENTS

90 Seconds to Calm: Your Breath Remote Control   iii

1   We Are Stressed Out   1

2   Chronic Stress is Killing Us   23

3   Escaping Reality – Unhealthy Numbing Tactics   43

4   The Science of Breath   55

5   The Mind, Body, and Breath Connection   85

6   Breath: The Silent Healer Within   129

7   The Art of Breath: Exploring Techniques for Wellness   163

8   Integrating Breath into Daily Life   193

9   Inner Calm is a Breath Away   223

Resources   235

ACKNOWLEDGMENTS

I wish to thank all of the people brave enough to try out Breathwork to change their lives for the better. Your inspirational words and testimonials emphasize the importance of this work. Thank you to Bill Walsh with Powerteam International for encouraging me to embrace success as my outcome. Thank you Angel Tuccy for holding my hand throughout the entire book-writing process and introducing me to NeedAGuest and podcasting. Thank you Caitlin Nisos and Ann Raines for reading, editing, and contributing to the many draft versions along the way and helping create this final version seeking to help people everywhere. Thank you Tammy De Mizra and all the members of The OST for your encouragement and having faith in me even when I didn't. Thank you Michael Neeley for perfectly timed formatting help. Thank you Brian Kelly with BreathMasters and Steven Jaggers with Somatiq who are pioneers in this field and have taught me so much. A big thank you to my loving husband, Chad May – your support means the world to me. Thank you to all of the many people who helped this book become a reality but are not mentioned here. You are in my heart even if your name is not on this page. Thank you all. I am forever grateful.

Disclaimer

Although I am a board-certified physician, I am not your physician. Before undertaking any new physical routine, starting a medication or stopping one, it is always advisable to discuss the changes you are considering with your personal physician first. To the best of my knowledge, what I offer in the following pages is true and written with the best of intentions. However, individual circumstances and responses can vary widely, and the information provided here may not be appropriate for everyone.

The techniques and advice provided in this book are not a substitute for professional medical advice, diagnosis, or treatment. Always seek the advice of your physician or other qualified health providers with any questions you may have regarding a medical condition. If you experience any discomfort or adverse effects from the practices suggested in this book, discontinue immediately and consult your healthcare provider.

By following the information in this book, you agree to assume full responsibility for your own health and well-being. The author and publisher disclaim any liability for any direct, indirect, incidental, or consequential damages resulting from the use of the information provided.

Also, if you would like to verify my credentials, I have recently remarried and now am using the name Dr. Jeannie May. My medical license and credentialing can be found under my previous name "Jean Lessly, M.D." For more information visit TheBreathMD.com

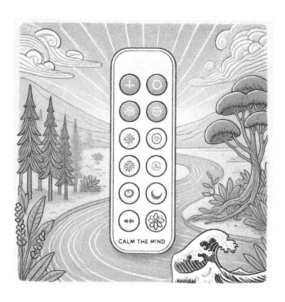

90 SECONDS TO CALM:
YOUR BREATH REMOTE CONTROL

Did you know that you can reset your emotional state in as little as 90 seconds by using only your breath? You have your own remote control to inner calm right under your nose. Let's try it out.

1. Inhale: Breathe in slowly and deeply through your nose for a count of 4 seconds.

2. Hold: Hold your breath for a count of 4 seconds.

3. Exhale: Exhale slowly and completely through your mouth or nose for a count of 6 seconds.

4. Repeat: Inhale again and repeat the above process for at least 90 seconds or keep going until you feel calmer.

This simple breathing pattern signals to your nervous system that "everything is ok – I am safe" and you can rest and relax. The best thing is you can do it anywhere, anytime absolutely free.

CHAPTER 1
WE ARE STRESSED OUT

"Stress is like a rocking chair. It gives you something to do, but it doesn't get you anywhere."

– Unknown

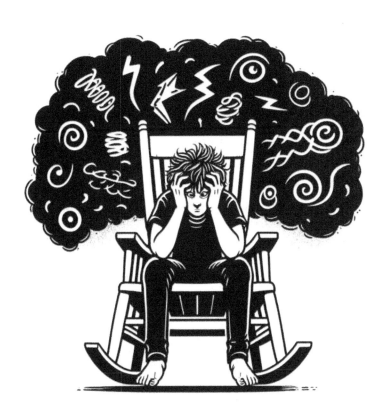

Navigating Stress: A Breath at a Time

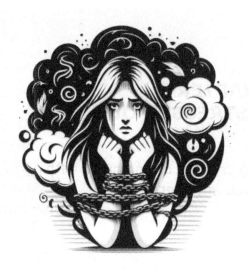

Are you a hostage to stress? I was. My entire identity was wrapped up in a state of chronic stress. Every moment was filled with this anxious feeling of being forever behind and overwhelmed. This was how I existed in the world, and I didn't think it could be any other way until the power of the breath changed my life. With this book, I am hoping it can change yours too.

Chronic stress is a silent killer, sneaking into our lives through the back door of modern living. It is the constant hum of anxiety, the weight of responsibility, and the pressure to perform. It is the sleepless nights, the racing thoughts, and the feeling of being stuck in overdrive. But beneath the surface, stress is wreaking havoc on our bodies. It is suppressing our immune system, fueling inflammation, and hijacking our hormonal balance. It is no wonder exhaustion and overwhelm are so common.

But what if we could break free from this cycle of stress and tap into a deeper sense of calm, clarity, and vitality? What if we could use our breath to reboot our nervous system to calm down and awaken our full potential? It turns out we can. We simply need to know how.

Welcome to the most intimate and powerful relationship we will ever have—the one with our breath. In a world where chronic stress has become the norm, our bodies are paying the price. We are constantly on edge, our minds racing, and our health is suffering as a result. But what if we had a remote control to calm the storm within? What if, with each breath, we could dial down the stress, quiet the mind, and reset our body's natural state of balance and well-being? The truth is, we do. The key to unlocking a life of calm and resilience is right under our nose.

Our breath is the ultimate remote control, waiting to be discovered and harnessed. In the pages that follow, we will embark on a journey to explore the transformative power of conscious breathing and how it can be the game-changer in our quest for inner calm, resilience, and vibrant health. Together, we will delve into the science and practice of Breathwork, uncovering the secrets to a life less burdened by stress and more filled with peace and vitality. Get ready to begin this journey toward a breath-centered, stress-free life.

The Modern Epidemic of Stress and Its Impact on Health

We all know stress is a major problem in our lives today. It is an epidemic affecting most of us and making us live with constant feelings of worry and overwhelm – but stress is not just a feeling. It can actually harm our bodies and make us sick.

In today's fast-paced world, stress seems to be everywhere. From school deadlines and work pressures to family responsibilities and social expectations, there's no shortage of things that can cause stress in our lives. While some stress is normal and even helpful in certain situations, too much of it can take a serious toll on our health and well-being.

Most of us have felt stress at one time or another. It simply seems to be a condition of modern times. Technology was supposed to make our lives easier, but now we are connected all the time and suffer from information overload leading to feelings of being overwhelmed which can cause total burnout. For example, it used to be when we mailed a letter, we had no choice but to wait for a response. Now with the internet, texts, social media, and emails, there is no waiting time. Something is always demanding our immediate attention and awaiting our response. The pace of the world has seemingly increased, and we keep running faster and faster to keep up. Stress is getting the best of us.

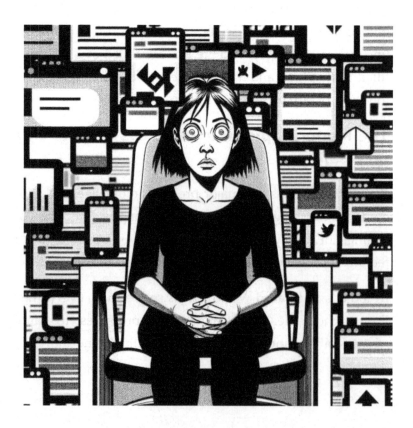

According to the World Health Organization (WHO), stress is considered the "health epidemic of the 21st century." It affects people of all ages, genders, and socioeconomic statuses. Up to 63% of US workers are ready to quit their jobs because of stress. The American Psychological Association (APA) estimates that workplace stress costs the US economy over $500 billion yearly.

Stress is not limited to the United States or even to developed countries for that matter. Stress is affecting the entire world. The Global Organization for Stress found that developing countries are experiencing increased stress levels as a result of rapid urbanization, economic instability, and social change. Stress is everywhere.

Chronic Stress and Our Health

When we experience stress, our body triggers a sympathetic nervous system response and goes into "fight or flight" mode, releasing hormones like adrenaline and cortisol to help us deal with the perceived threat. This response can be useful in short bursts, allowing us to react quickly to danger or challenges. However, when stress becomes chronic – lingering for weeks, months, or even years – it can wreak havoc on our bodies.

Chronic stress has been linked to a wide range of health problems, including heart disease, high blood pressure, obesity, diabetes, depression, and anxiety. It weakens our immune system, making us more susceptible to infections and illnesses. Stress can disrupt our sleep patterns, leaving us feeling tired and irritable. It can even accelerate the aging process, contributing to wrinkles, gray hair, and other signs of premature aging. The American Psychological Association found that 70% of Americans reported experiencing at least one symptom of stress in the past month.

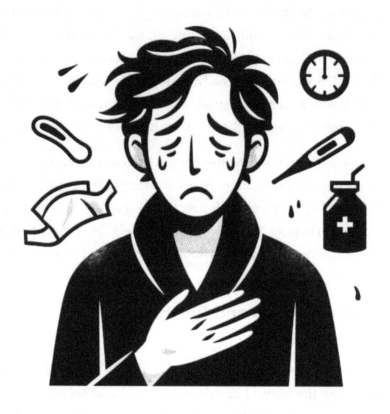

Most concerning of all is the impact of chronic stress on our mental health. It can lead to feelings of sadness, hopelessness, and despair, eroding our sense of happiness and fulfillment. It can impair our cognitive functioning, making it difficult to concentrate, remember things, and make decisions. It affects our relationships, contributing to conflicts with loved ones resulting in feelings of loneliness and isolation.

In short, stress is more than just a minor inconvenience – it's a serious threat to our health and well-being. And with the pace of modern life showing no signs of slowing down, it's more important than ever to find effective ways to manage and reduce our stress levels. Our lives depend on it.

The Breath-Stress Connection

When we are stressed, our breathing changes. It becomes shallow, rapid, and erratic. This triggers a cascade of physiological responses that prepare our body for "fight or flight" behavior. Our heart rate increases, blood pressure rises, and our nervous system goes into hyperalert mode. This response was designed to save our lives in emergency situations, but when it becomes chronic, it starts to destroy our health.

The way we breathe is a reflection of how we live. If we find ourselves holding our breath, we are likely holding back, controlling, and diverting energy from our own creativity and even our most important relationships. The simple act of breathing could be the most powerful tool to transform our interaction with stress and anxiety.

Imagine waking up each day feeling energized, focused, and at peace. We can harness the power of our breath to shift from surviving to thriving in a world filled with stress and uncertainty. The answer to managing chronic stress is not another app or gadget, 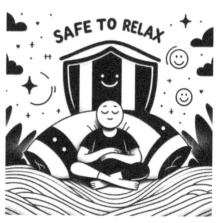 but rather a deeper understanding of our own breath. By changing our breathing patterns, we can signal to our body that it is safe to relax, calm down, and return to balance. This is where conscious breathing comes in—a powerful tool for optimizing our nervous system, calming our minds, and restoring our natural state of well-being.

In the following chapters, we will explore the science behind Breathwork, the different techniques for harnessing its power, and the transformative stories of those who have used it to overcome stress, anxiety, and burnout. We will also dive into the practical applications of Breathwork, from improving sleep and focus to enhancing creativity and productivity. Get ready to unlock the full potential of your breath and discover a life of calm, clarity, and vitality.

The Overlooked Power of Breath in Managing Stress

With chronic stress eroding our very quality of life, becoming familiar with the power of breath has never been more important. Our breath is something we often take for granted. It's automatic – we don't have to think about it. But what if I told you that by paying attention to your breath and learning to regulate it, you could unlock a whole world of benefits for your mental and physical health?

Breathing may seem simple and mundane, but our breath is actually a powerful tool for managing stress and promoting relaxation. By learning to regulate our breathing, we can activate the body's natural relaxation response, calming our nervous system and soothing our mind.

Most of us don't realize how powerful our breath can be in dealing with the stresses agitating our minds and bodies. It's like having a remote control to bring inner calm whenever we need it. When we are stressed, our breathing tends to become shallow and rapid. This is part of the body's natural response to stress – to prepare us for action. But the problem is that when we breathe this way for too long, it can actually make our stress worse. It's like pouring fuel on the fire. Luckily, the good news is that we can break the cycle by consciously changing the way we breathe. By taking slow, deep breaths into our diaphragm, we can send a signal to our brain that everything is okay – that we are safe and there's no need to be in "fight or flight" response anymore.

Healthy Breathing

Most people believe that because our breathing is automatic, we are automatically breathing healthily - but nothing could be further from the truth. Most of us are conditioned to be rapid, shallow chest-breathers. Some of us even breathe through our mouths most of the time which causes even greater problems. The act of breathing rapidly and shallowly into our chest activates the "fight or flight" branch of our nervous system. The way most of us breathe, actually increases stress and anxiety without our even being aware we are doing it.

If you want to observe a healthy breather, then simply observe a baby breathing. A baby takes a very slow breath in through the nose and pulls the breath down into its belly. We can see it's belly rise and fall. It is a very natural process. That is a healthy breath. But most people as a result of the food that we eat, the environment we live in, our sedentary lifestyle, our chronic stress, and anxiety level are 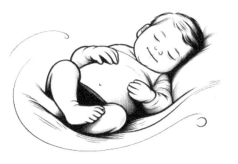 overbreathing using shallow, rapid chest-breaths. Many people snore and have sleep apnea and breathe through their mouths as a result. All of this activates the "fight or flight" nervous system and puts us constantly on edge.

Remote Control to Inner Calm

Right now, we have the power with our breath to reset our mood and decrease stress in less than 90 seconds. Most of us have no idea we have this control. This is the magic of Breathwork. Our nervous system has multiple fluctuations often occurring within minutes which are directly tied to our emotional system. Often we get into these emotional states, and we don't know how to get out of them. Most people simply wait helplessly for their emotional state to change. It doesn't have to be this way. Breathwork is a tool that allows us to up-regulate, down-regulate, or simply balance our nervous system in mere seconds without complicated or expensive machines. How great is that!

Breathing is the only thing within our autonomic nervous system that we can control. We cannot control our heart rate, blood pressure, digestion, or the thousands of other processes that are happening in our bodies under autonomic nervous control—except for our breath. We can immediately affect the quality of our nervous system by shifting from these fast, shallow upper chest breaths to slow, deep breaths into the belly. When we take deep breaths, it automatically activates the "rest and digest" side of the nervous system, known as the parasympathetic nervous system. When we control our breathing, then our mind and our body will respond and relax.

The Box Breath

Let's try it. Take one hand and put it on your belly. Now take a nice slow deep breath in through your nose very slowly and gently all the way down to your lower abdomen. You should feel your belly expand on the inhale. Then exhale your breath completely either through your nose or through your mouth and repeat one more time.

Next let's try the Box Breath by taking a breath in for a count of four, hold your breath for a count of four, exhale for a count of four, hold for a count of four and then repeat. This is called a Box Breath and it does wonders for decreasing stress and relieving anxiety. The incredible thing is you can do the Box Breath in a crowd without anyone even knowing you are doing it. You have your own remote control for stress using only your breath.

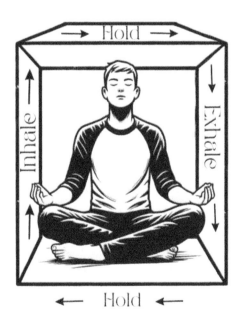

Deep breathing activates the body's relaxation response, triggering the release of feel good hormones like serotonin and endorphins. It slows down our heart rate, lowers our blood pressure, and relaxes our muscles. It also calms the mind, quieting the chatter of anxious thoughts and helping us feel more centered and grounded.

Breathwork Availability

But perhaps the most remarkable thing about Breathwork is its accessibility. Unlike other stress relief techniques that require special equipment or training, all we need to practice Breathwork is our own breath and conscious awareness. It is free, portable, and available to everyone 24/7. Whether we are old or young, fit or out of shape, experienced at meditation or brand-new to the practice, there's something here for everybody.

Think about it – it's like carrying around a powerful stress relief tool in our pocket wherever we go. When we are stuck in traffic, waiting in line at the grocery store, or dealing with a difficult situation at work, we can always turn to our breath for support. We are able to regulate ourselves anywhere, anytime.

And the best part? The more we practice, the more effective it becomes. Over time, we will develop a greater awareness of our breath and its connection to our emotions. We will learn to recognize the signs of stress in our body and respond to them with calm and clarity.

My Story: Stressful Chaos to Breathwork Bliss

Of all the difficulties of my life, nothing has been more challenging than the dark clouds of stress, always sprinkling if not outright pouring on me throughout my life. Stress was all I knew. It was the background noise against which my life played out. Stress was always there. I felt helpless to make it go away, all the while yearning for serenity but not knowing if peace was possible for me, much less how to get it.

My overachieving began in grade school as I strived to make good grades, thinking this would make me worthy of affection and appreciation. Much of my stress was self-induced. In fact, I became addicted to stress. When things would get too quiet, I would find a way to increase the pressure cooker of my life.

Having gone to public school in Tennessee through the eighth grade, I intensified my stress by transferring to a private high school on scholarship the first year it went coed. I was one of 41 girls in a school of 650 boys at The Baylor School in Chattanooga. We were featured in the newspapers and TV news as "The Fabulous 41" with tremendous pressure placed on us to succeed. The transition from public school to private school was incredibly difficult. At the time, public schools in Tennessee were ranked 49th in the nation (we were always grateful for Mississippi for taking last place). I had to study in a way I had never studied before in order to obtain the straight A's I demanded of myself. Luckily, it taught me a self-discipline that made college easy.

At Vassar College, I majored in political science with the intention of becoming an attorney. In 1990, I continued my self-induced stress by traveling for my junior year abroad to Moscow, USSR, two weeks after Gorbachev had been kidnapped following an attempted coup.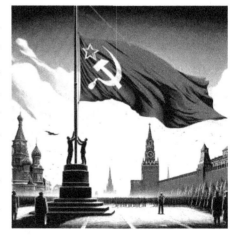
The USSR was falling apart. In fact, I watched the flag change from the vast, powerful, and feared Soviet Union down to the single country of Russia on Christmas day 1990. Uncertainty was everywhere and seemed to be the only thing left after the collapse of the Soviet Union. The entire country was stressed.

Meanwhile, there were tremendous shortages in food and supplies. People would see long lines and stand in them just in case there was something good they could buy at the end of it. The hospitals had no anesthesia, pain medications, or surgical supplies. I watched a medical procedure where the patient bit his hand to endure the pain and an old woman died unattended in a hospital hallway. I witnessed the fear of the people around me lost in a sea of anxiety—unsure from where next week's food would come. The money exchange rate was completely out of whack, and for the first time in my life, I was rich. A McDonald's had just opened up, but one Big Mac was an average Russian's monthly salary so only foreigners and the Russian mafia could afford it.

I attended MGIMO, the most prestigious international law school in the Soviet Union which was actually a training ground for future KGB agents. I hated law school because the people were so fake, and it always seemed like they were spying on me. Luckily, I was living with a family on the outskirts of Moscow and became friends with many of the local people in my neighborhood. One of the boys there was attending medical school, so on my off days from law school, I accompanied him. Russians were not accustomed to Westerners at this time and welcomed me as an interesting oddity. It was in Russia that I realized I was not destined for law and decided I wanted to become a doctor. The law was about representing clients whether they were guilty or not. In medicine, what is best for the patient is always the right answer—or at least it should be.

When I returned to the United States, I had not taken a single college science class. Originally, I considered going to veterinary school, but the prerequisites were much more difficult. At the time, there were only four science classes required to apply to medical school. I started taking those classes immediately and ultimately graduated Phi Beta Kappa with a political science degree. However, I still had to wait another year after graduation to complete my requirements to enter medical school. I had a 4.0 GPA in my four science classes and did very well on the MCATs but was waitlisted to the top schools because of my limited science background. With all of the changes in my educational path, peace, calm and serenity were nowhere in sight.

As I waited to see if medical school was a possibility, I went back to Moscow to visit my friends. While I was there, being a glutton for stress and pressure, I went solo skydiving for the first time with only 30 minutes of instruction in Russian (which I did not understand) prior to jumping. Although I would not 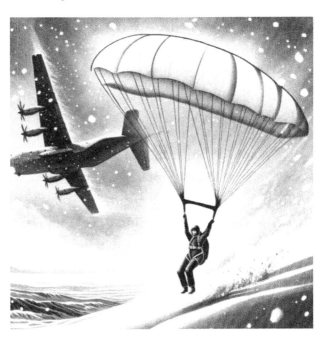 repeat such behavior, I do believe the picture of me in the snow with the parachute behind me helped me get off the waitlist and into Washington University School of Medicine in St. Louis, then ranked third in the nation overall and number one for student selectivity.

Medical school was a level of stress I had never experienced before in my entire life. I was taking advanced biochemistry even though I had never taken introductory biochemistry. At the same time, I was in a class with the top ranked students in the country. Needless to say, I almost flunked out my first year. After much perseverance—and a whole lot of tutoring—I passed the first two years of the classroom and excelled in the clinicals, graduating in the top half of my class.

I didn't think anything could be harder than medical school, but I hadn't been through residency yet. To become a doctor you must complete four years of college, four years of medical school, followed by a year-long internship, and then by 2 to 3 more years of residency – and I added on a year fellowship for a little more stress. If I'd had any idea how incredibly difficult it is to become a doctor, I don't think I would have done it. Don't get me wrong, now that I've made it, I'm glad that I did, but I can't imagine doing it again.

My years of Internal Medicine residency at Vanderbilt University Medical Center were among the hardest of my life. Although things are very different now, we would work 120 hours a week while spending the night in the hospital every 2nd to 4th day. In the intensive care units we would work 28 hours in the hospital, 20 hours off, and then 28 hours on alternating shifts for six weeks. I once worked a 54 hour shift without going home. I would literally bite my tongue and pinch my skin to stay awake. Multiple times I fell asleep standing up—something I had not even realized was possible for non-horses.

In many ways, residency was an obstacle meant to scare people into quitting. Indeed the stress was so much for many that they did drop out—I would have been one of them if I had not been over $200,000 in debt from medical school and saw no way out. People quit not because they were not capable of being good doctors, but because the environment was simply too stressful. To make things even more difficult, I was pregnant with my oldest daughter during my third year of residency. To say I was absolutely exhausted and stressed is an understatement.

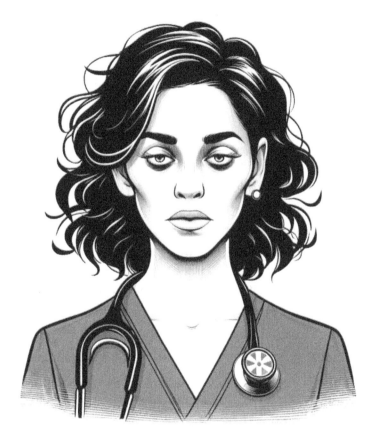

My addiction to stress didn't stop there. Throughout my 25 plus years of medical practice, I frequently worked at least five different jobs at a time. If I wasn't pushing myself to a point of exhaustion while putting out patient emergencies, taking care of routine patients, running a medical business, while raising my children, I wouldn't know what to do with myself. I even got board-certified with four different certifications including

Internal Medicine, Geriatrics, Hospice and Palliative Medicine, and Addiction Medicine. Stress was my constant companion.

Looking back, when I think about all the opportunities and adventures that I have had, I can say that I could have experienced so much more joy and laughter in the moment, but I was overwhelmed with so much anxiety and stress that my memories of my past are more of the fear I experienced rather than the happy times of my life. If it weren't for stress and my resultant perception of the world, I could have enjoyed the journey rather than always pressing the present trying to arrive in the future.

Part of me knew that something had to change because I could not keep up this pace forever. In my effort to take care of others, I had neglected myself and had chronic pain, depression, anxiety, high blood pressure, and high cholesterol as a result. It hurt to move and just getting out of bed in the morning was becoming more and more difficult.

As part of my continuing education, I decided to investigate Somatic Release Breathwork as I thought it would help my patients in Addiction Medicine with their anxiety. It turned out to be something completely different than I had anticipated. In one 90 minute session, I experienced what felt like five years of talk therapy. Years of unprocessed emotion and trapped trauma left me, and I felt better than I could have imagined. The amazing thing is that the healing lasted. I was so impressed by this new healing therapy that I plunged into learning all that I possibly could. Here was a way to get to the root of so many problems. I have discovered a significant number of my addiction patients do not use drugs to get high, they're using drugs to get numb. Breathwork was a way without pharmaceuticals to create lasting change in healing. And there are no side effects, very unlike the medications I prescribe. It is simply breathing, something we have been doing all of our lives. The breath has a magic power to heal, and my goal is to bring it to the world.

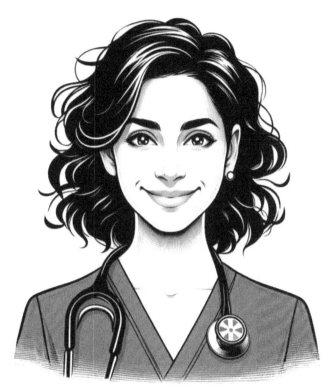

Breathe Better, Feel Better

In this book, we will explore how breathing can be a super tool for managing stress and feeling better throughout our bodies and minds, without needing to adjust our external circumstances. We will look at simple techniques anyone can use and how they work. My goal is to help increase understanding of the amazing potential of our breath and how to use it to live a happier, healthier life.

Breathing is something we do without even thinking about it. It's a natural, automatic process that keeps us alive. But what many people don't realize is that our breath has incredible power to influence our physical and mental well-being.

But this book isn't just about theory – I will also provide practical, hands-on techniques that can be used right away to harness the power of our breath. From simple exercises that focus on deep, diaphragmatic breathing to more advanced practices like pranayama and mindfulness meditation, we will discover a variety of tools to help us cultivate a more mindful relationship with our breath.

In this book, we will explore a variety of breath work techniques designed to help us manage stress and cultivate inner peace. From simple breathing exercises we can do in just a few minutes a day to more advanced practices that also deepen our connection to our breath, there's something here for everyone.

My goal is to demystify Breathwork and make it accessible to people from all walks of life. I want to show that we don't need to be a yoga guru or meditation master to benefit from the power of our breath. All it takes is a little curiosity and a willingness to try something new.

Throughout this book, we will explore the fascinating science behind the breath-body connection and discover practical techniques for harnessing the power of breath to reduce stress and improve overall well-being. From simple breathing exercises we can do anytime, anywhere, to mindfulness practices that help us stay present and grounded, we will cover a wide range of strategies for incorporating Breathwork into our life.

As we journey through this book, I encourage an open-minded approach with a spirit of curiosity. Experiment with different techniques and see what works best. Remember that Breathwork is a personal journey, and there's no one-size-fits-all approach. Trust the body's wisdom while exploring the transformative potential of our breath.

This book's goal is to empower us with the knowledge and skills we need to take control of our stress and live a happier, healthier life. This shift and practice may start in the response to immediate stressors and can develop into ongoing preventative self-care. By the time we reach the end of this book, my hope is that we will not only have a deeper understanding of the incredible power of our breath but also a newfound sense of empowerment to use it as a tool for healing, transformation, and self-discovery. So take a deep breath, relax, and let's embark on this journey together.

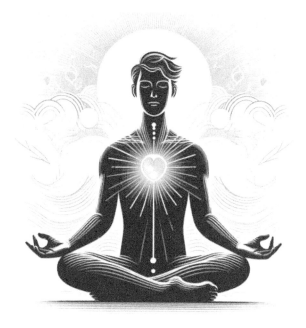

2
CHRONIC STRESS IS KILLING US

"Stress is the trash of modern life - we all generate it, but if you don't dispose of it properly, it will pile up and overtake your life."

- Danzae Pace

Stress: What Is It Really?

Feeling stressed is something we have all experienced. It's like our body goes into full alert mode. Our stomach feels all twisted up, our chest feels tight like someone's squeezing it, and our shoulders tense up so much they practically touch our ears. We might notice our heart beating faster, our breath coming quicker, and our mind racing with worries. It's like our whole body is ready to fight something, even if there's nothing there. Our body is preparing for battle, even if we are just sitting at our desk or lying in bed.

Stress can affect everyone differently. Some people might get headaches or stomachaches, while others might feel tired or irritable. But no matter how it appears, stress is our body's way of telling us that something isn't quite right. It's like a warning sign that we need to take a step back and figure out how to cope.

Sometimes, stress comes from big things, like a difficult project at work or a fight with a friend. But other times, it can creep up on us for no apparent reason, making us feel anxious and overwhelmed. Being constantly stressed can become our normal state—but it's not a healthy way to live.

Sheila's Story: The Toll of Chronic Stress on Health

Sheila was a high-functioning attorney with a relentless drive for success. Her dedication and hard work earned her accolades and a prestigious position at a top law firm. However, this success came at a high cost. Sheila often found herself working late into the night, skipping meals, and sacrificing sleep to meet the demands of her job. The stress from her high-pressure environment began to take a toll on her health.

Unbeknownst to her colleagues, Sheila was battling systemic lupus erythematous, an autoimmune condition that causes joint pain, rashes, and severe fatigue. The chronic stress and exhaustion from her work significantly weakened her immune system, triggering severe flare-ups. Each time she pushed herself too hard, her body responded with debilitating pain and inflammation.

This led to a vicious cycle. Sheila would overwork herself, leading to a suppressed immune system and subsequent flare-ups of her lupus. The pain and fatigue would force her to take extended medical leave,

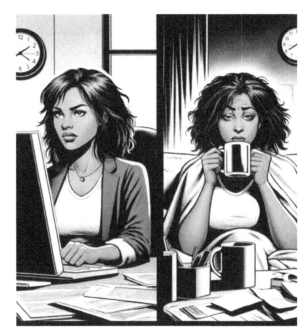

during which she would focus on resetting her nervous system and recovering her strength. Once she felt better, she would dive back into her demanding workload, only for the cycle to repeat itself.

Sheila's story highlights how chronic stress can severely impact physical health. The constant pressure and lack of self-care led to a negative feedback loop, where stress exacerbated her painful lupus, causing repeated health crises. Despite her professional success, Sheila's health suffered immensely, affecting her overall quality of life.

Tribal Life and Stress

Understanding stress starts with thinking about how humans have changed over time. Let's go back to when our ancestors lived in tribes. In those times, life was pretty simple: either things were going well or they weren't. When things were tough, it was usually because something threatened survival, such as not having enough food, an aggressive wild animal, a drought, or a neighboring tribe causing trouble. These threats were clear and immediate, activating our ancestors' fight-or-flight response, a survival mechanism to respond to immediate dangers.

When there was a real danger, everyone could see it. And when that happened, everyone in the tribe worked together to stay

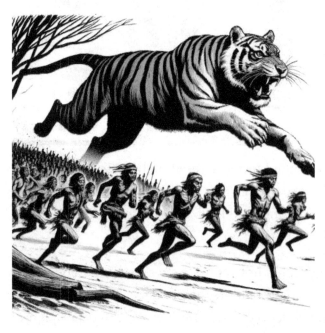

safe. This communal response not only increased chances of survival but also fostered strong social bonds, crucial for the well-being and cohesion of the group. These social bonds and cooperative behaviors were adaptations that helped our ancestors survive and thrive.

Now let's look at today. When can we say we're not worried? It seems like there's always something bothering us, even if it's not a big deal. But unlike in the past, these worries aren't usually about staying alive. We are worried about work, money, relationships, health, the environment, political uncertainty, our kids, our parents, and a million other things. We are always dealing with some level of stress, even if it's not life-or-death. These chronic stressors are often less immediate and tangible than the threats our ancestors faced, but they still activate our stress response system as if it were life or death. This mismatch between the types of stressors we face today and those our brains evolved to handle emergencies is a significant issue.

Our brains are still wired like those of our ancestors. We're built to deal with immediate dangers, not the constant, low-level stress of modern life. Our brains haven't caught up with how the world has changed. This mismatch between our ancient instincts and our modern lives is a key factor of why stress is such a big problem today.

Our stress response system, optimized for the sporadic and acute threats of the ancestral environment, is now constantly triggered by the chronic, varied, and often abstract stressors of modern life. This constant activation of the stress response system can lead to a variety of health problems, including anxiety, depression, cardiovascular disease, and weakened immune function.

Consider the example of a dog scared of thunder. Many animals, including dogs, have a natural fear of thunderstorms or fireworks. This fear can cause them to exhibit signs of anxiety, such as trembling, hiding, or destructive behavior. The loud noises trigger a fear response meant to protect them from potential threats in the wild. We don't judge the dog for its fear;

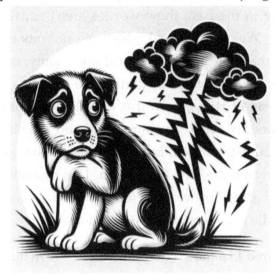

instead, we recognize it, acknowledging that this fear is a product of its instincts.

This understanding of instinct and its forgiveness can be applied to patterns of unresolved anxiety and baseless fears in our own modern lives to increase self-compassion and discernment. It is as if it is thundering all the time around us, and we struggle to distinguish between what is our baseline and what is all the noise on top of that. We should not be afraid or stressed, but we are. Our ancient instincts struggle to keep up with the complexities of modern society, where threats are not always immediate or physical. This mismatch between our evolutionary heritage and our current environment is a key factor in why stress is such a pervasive problem today.

Suppression of Emotions Adds to Our Stress

In our Western culture, there's often a push to hide our feelings. From a young age, we're told to "stop crying" or that it's not okay to show anger or fear. This conditioning makes us uncomfortable when these emotions surface, so we try to bury them deep inside, hoping they'll disappear on their own.

But guess what? Ignoring our emotions doesn't make them go away. In fact, it takes a lot of effort to keep them down. Staying numb is an active process. It's like trying to hold a beach ball underwater—eventually, it is going to pop up. We distract ourselves with things like TV, movies, alcohol, or drugs to keep those emotions buried. We scroll endlessly on our phones, hoping to avoid facing what's really bothering us. But deep down, the stress and unhappiness lingers.

Why do we go to such lengths to stay numb? Because we have rarely been given permission to feel. Society tells us to toughen up, to put on a brave face, that it's not okay to feel sad, angry, hurt, or afraid. Suppressing these emotions only leads to more pain in the long run.

The Stress of Sudden Trauma

When we sense danger, our body reacts without even thinking about it – we might want to fight, runaway, or freeze in place. It is instinctual. This quick response is important because it helps keep us safe. Our reaction is automatic and necessary for survival. The body gets a sudden burst of energy to prepare for whatever we need to do. This reaction is something we have inherited from our ancestors who needed to survive in the wild. It is our built-in alarm system, helping us deal with tough situations and making sure we are ready to handle anything that comes our way.

Let's look at an example. If someone breaks into our home with a gun, our body floods with stress hormones such as adrenaline and cortisol, and we act without thinking. Instinct takes over. We fight, run away, or freeze. It is automatic as our body focuses on keeping us safe to survive the threat. We are not thinking. We are not processing our emotions. We are in the moment, trying to survive.

If we fight or flee, that revved-up energy gets used. But if we freeze, that energy stays trapped inside us. Now, freezing isn't a 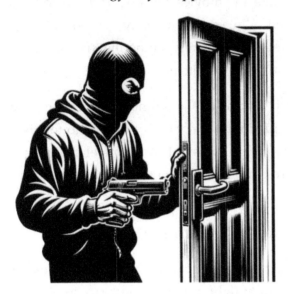 bad thing. It's a natural survival instinct that keeps us safe in dangerous situations where fighting or fleeing are not an option— sometimes freezing is the best choice we have. The problem comes afterwards, after the danger has passed. Animals in the wild shake off that pent-up energy after a freeze event, signaling to their bodies that the threat is gone. They're safe. Humans, on the other hand, often suppress that energy, leading to trapped trauma in our bodies that can cause chronic stress and a feeling of being unsafe. We may carry this trapped trauma for years to come and it can affect our every interaction in the world.

What's so strange is that we might not even remember the traumas that triggered our lingering stress and anxiety. It could be something as simple as a childhood injury or a forgotten dental procedure. Events no longer in our conscious memory can negatively affect how we interact with our world as we feel helpless to control them.

Many people turn to talk therapy to address the mental side of trauma, and while it can be helpful, it doesn't always ease the deep-seated stress, anxiety, and depression. To truly heal, we need to release the emotions we've been holding. This lets our nervous system know that we are safe now—the danger has passed.

It is important to give ourselves permission to feel. We need to acknowledge our emotions, whether they're positive or negative, and allow ourselves to experience them fully. This doesn't mean dwelling on our problems endlessly, but rather, allowing ourselves to process and release whatever we're feeling.

By giving ourselves permission to feel, we can free ourselves from the burden of suppressed emotions and live more authentically in the moment, rather than being caught in the past or the future.

Do You Have Stress?

Stress is something we all experience at some point in our lives. It's the body's natural response to demands or threats, and it can affect us physically, emotionally, and mentally. When we are stressed, our body is basically 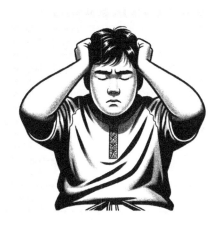 in a state of high alert all the time. It is like our body is constantly on edge, ready to react to any potential threat. This can be really exhausting and can take a toll on both our physical and mental health. But how do we know if we are experiencing stress? Here are some common symptoms to look out for:

Muscle Tension

When we are stressed, our muscles tend to tighten up, leading to tension headaches, neck and shoulder pain, and overall discomfort.

Anxiety

Feelings of worry, nervousness, or unease are common signs of stress. We may find it difficult to relax or feel constantly tense.

Depression

Chronic stress can take a toll on our mood, leading to feelings of sadness, hopelessness, or emptiness. We may lose interest in activities we once enjoyed and have trouble concentrating.

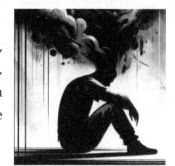

Digestive Problems

Stress can wreak havoc on our digestive system, leading to symptoms like stomach cramps, bloating, diarrhea, or constipation.

Weight Gain or Weight Loss

Stress can affect our appetite and eating habits, leading to changes in weight. Some people may turn to food for comfort, leading to weight gain, while others may lose their appetite and shed pounds unintentionally.

Insomnia

Difficulty falling asleep or staying asleep is a common symptom of stress. Racing thoughts and worries can keep us awake at night, leading to sleep disturbances and fatigue during the day.

Pain

Stress can exacerbate existing pain conditions or cause new ones to develop. Headaches, back pain, and muscle aches are common complaints among stressed individuals.

High Blood Pressure

Prolonged stress can contribute to high blood pressure, increasing the risk of heart disease, stroke, and other cardiovascular problems.

High Blood Sugar

Stress can also affect blood sugar levels, particularly in individuals with diabetes or pre-diabetes. Fluctuations in blood sugar can lead to mood swings, fatigue, and other complications.

Addictions

Some people turn to substances like cigarettes, alcohol, or drugs to cope with stress. Others may develop addictive behaviors such as overeating, compulsive shopping, video games, or gambling as a way to escape their problems temporarily.

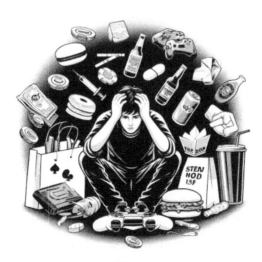

These symptoms of stress may vary in intensity and duration depending on the individual and the level of stress they're experiencing. While occasional stress is a normal part of life, chronic or excessive stress can have serious consequences for our health and well-being.

Chronic Stress: The Silent Killer

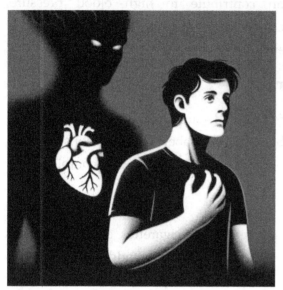

Chronic stress is like a silent thief that sneaks up on us and steals our health and well-being. Unlike acute stress, which is short-lived and easily identifiable, chronic stress can be harder to recognize because it often builds up slowly over time. When we are stressed out all the time, it can start to feel normal. We might not even realize how stressed we are until we start to notice the negative effects on our health and happiness. It's like the background noise that's always there, gradually wearing us down without our even realizing it. It is like a slow leak in the tire – it's not always obvious until it's too late.

One of the insidious things about chronic stress is that it can affect every aspect of our lives. It can impact our physical health and mental health while straining our relationships, causing conflicts with loved ones and feelings of isolation and loneliness.

It can even affect our work or school performance, making it difficult to concentrate, remember things, or make decisions.

Chronic stress can also shorten our lifespan, increasing our risk of premature death from heart disease, stroke, or other stress-related illnesses. In short, chronic stress is not something to be taken lightly—it's a serious threat to our health and longevity that requires attention and intervention.

Stress is Linked to Seven Leading Causes of Death

Chronic stress is linked to seven leading causes of death including: heart attack, stroke, cancer, lung disease, accidents, cirrhosis of the liver, and suicide. Stress can literally kill you. It affects every organ system and ultimately affects the very way we live our lives. Take a look at the following statistics regarding how chronic stress affects our bodies:

Cardiovascular Health

- Chronic stress increases the risk of heart disease by 40%.
- Stress contributes also to hypertension, with 33% of adults reporting high stress levels experiencing high blood pressure.
- Chronic stress is associated with elevated cholesterol levels and inflammation in the body which can damage the arteries, leading to conditions like heart attacks, strokes, and coronary artery disease.

Immune System

- Chronic stress weakens the immune system, making individuals more susceptible to infections, illnesses, and chronic diseases. Prolonged stress can impair the body's ability to fight off pathogens and heal from injuries, leading to frequent illnesses and prolonged recovery times.

- Chronic stress can worsen autoimmune diseases, such as rheumatoid arthritis and lupus.

Digestive System

- Stress can lead to gastrointestinal issues such as irritable bowel syndrome (IBS) with increased diarrhea or constipation, gastritis, ulcers, abdominal pain, and acid reflux.
- Chronic stress can disrupt the balance of gut bacteria, leading to digestive problems.
- Stress is a common trigger for flare-ups in conditions like Crohn's Disease and Ulcerative Colitis.

Mental Health Disorders

- Chronic stress is a significant risk factor for developing anxiety, depression, and other mental health conditions.
- Stress can affect neurotransmitter levels in the brain, alter mood-regulating hormones, and impair cognitive functioning, leading to emotional instability and psychological distress.
- Stress contributes to 70% of visits to primary care physicians.

Substance Abuse and Addiction

- Individuals with chronic stress are more likely to engage in substance abuse as a coping mechanism.
- Many people turn to substances like alcohol, tobacco, or drugs as a way to cope with stress and manage their emotions. Chronic stress can increase the risk of substance abuse and addiction by altering brain chemistry, impairing judgment and decision-making, and reinforcing addictive behaviors.

Brain Function

- Prolonged stress can lead to structural changes in the brain, particularly in areas associated with memory and emotion regulation.
- Chronic stress has been linked to an increased risk of neurodegenerative diseases like Alzheimer's Disease and other dementias.
- Stress impairs cognitive function, including memory, concentration, and decision-making abilities.

Sleep

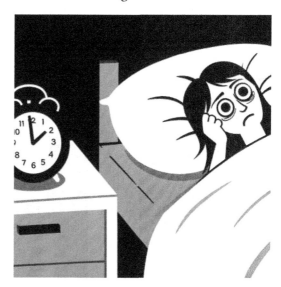

- Stress disrupts sleep patterns, with 45% of adults reporting that stress affects their sleep quality.
- Chronic stress can disrupt the body's natural sleep-wake cycle, leading to insomnia, restless sleep, and frequent awakenings during the night contributing to daytime fatigue and irritability.
- Sleep disturbances caused by stress can worsen existing health conditions.

Weight and Metabolism

- Stress contributes to weight gain, particularly around the abdominal area, increasing the risk of obesity and metabolic syndrome.

- Chronic stress can lead to unhealthy eating habits, such as emotional eating and cravings for high-fat and sugary foods.
- Stress-induced changes in metabolism can increase the risk of Type 2 Diabetes and insulin resistance.

Pain Perception

- Stress can heighten the perception of pain, increasing conditions such as migraines, fibromyalgia, and chronic back pain.
- Chronic stress can lead to muscle tension and worsen existing musculoskeletal conditions.

Skin Health

- Chronic stress can worsen skin conditions such as eczema, psoriasis, and acne.
- Stress hormones can increase oil production in the skin, leading to breakouts and acne flare-ups.

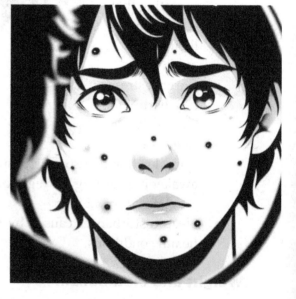

- Stress-induced inflammation can increase symptoms of chronic skin conditions and delay wound healing.

Reproductive Health

- Chronic stress can disrupt menstrual cycles and contribute to irregular periods and menstrual cramps.
- Stress can affect fertility by disrupting hormone levels and ovulation in women and sperm production in men.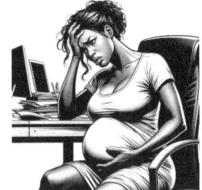
- Pregnant individuals experiencing high levels of stress are at increased risk of complications such as preterm birth and low birth weight as well as increased stress hormones in the baby.

Respiratory Health

- Stress can worsen respiratory conditions such as asthma, allergic reactions, and chronic obstructive pulmonary disease (COPD).
- Individuals with chronic stress may experience more frequent and severe asthma attacks.
- Stress-induced shallow breathing can increase respiratory symptoms and decrease lung function.

Endocrine System

- Chronic stress can throw hormone levels off balance, leading to conditions such as adrenal fatigue and thyroid disorders.
- Stress hormones like cortisol can disrupt insulin sensitivity, increasing the risk of Type 2 Diabetes.
- Stress-induced changes in hormone levels can impact reproductive health, metabolism, and energy levels.

Cancer Risk

- Chronic stress may contribute to cancer progression by suppressing the immune system and promoting inflammation.
- Stressful life events have been linked to an increased risk of developing certain types of cancer, including breast and colorectal cancers.

Eye Health

- Chronic stress can worsen eye conditions such as dry eye syndrome and eye twitching.
- Stress-induced tension in the muscles around the eyes can lead to headaches and eye strain.
- Stress may increase symptoms of vision disorders such as myopia and astigmatism.

Dental Health

- Chronic stress can contribute to oral health problems such as bruxism (teeth grinding) and temporomandibular joint (TMJ) disorders.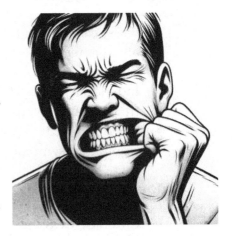
- Stress-induced changes in saliva production and composition can increase the risk of tooth decay and gum disease.

Hormonal Imbalance

- Chronic stress can disrupt the balance of sex hormones, leading to issues such as menstrual irregularities and decreased libido.

- Stress-induced changes in hormone levels can contribute to symptoms of menopause, such as hot flashes and mood swings.
- Hormonal imbalances caused by stress may increase the risk of conditions such as polycystic ovary syndrome (PCOS) and erectile dysfunction.

Inflammation

- Chronic stress triggers systemic inflammation, which is associated with an increased risk of chronic diseases such as cardiovascular disease and diabetes.
- Stress-induced inflammation can worsen symptoms of inflammatory conditions such as rheumatoid arthritis and inflammatory bowel disease.

Bone Health

- Chronic stress can weaken bones and increase the risk of osteoporosis and fractures.
- Stress-induced changes in hormone levels can disrupt bone remodeling processes, leading to decreased bone density.

Quality of Life

- Chronic stress can significantly impact quality of life, leading to decreased enjoyment of activities and social withdrawal.
- Stress-related fatigue and burnout can interfere with work performance and relationships.
- Stress management interventions can improve overall quality of life and well-being.

Long-Term Health Consequences

- Chronic stress is associated with an increased risk of premature death, with stress-related conditions contributing to a reduction in life expectancy.
- The cumulative effects of chronic stress over time can lead to a decline in overall health and functional status.

Stress is a prevalent issue in today's world, impacting many aspects of our lives. We often overlook the constant pressure we face each day, but chronic stress can have severe consequences for our health. It's essential to recognize the signs and take steps to manage stress effectively. Ignoring chronic stress can lead to serious health problems and even be life-threatening. By acknowledging the impact of stress on our well-being and adopting healthy coping mechanisms, we can lessen its harmful effects and improve our overall quality of life. Don't underestimate the importance of addressing stress—it's not just a minor inconvenience but a significant factor in our long-term health and happiness. It can have serious health consequences and left unchecked, can be deadly. Luckily, the power of our breath offers us a solution.

3
ESCAPING REALITY – UNHEALTHY NUMBING TACTICS

"It's not the load that breaks you down, it's the way you carry it."

- Lou Holtz

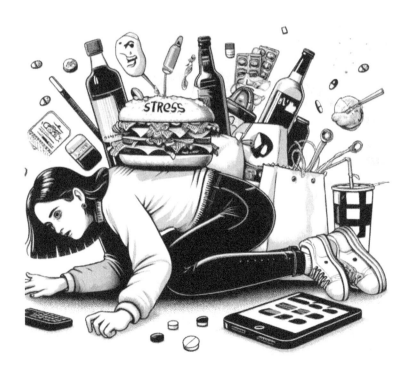

Robert's Story: A Day of Escaping Reality

Robert stood in front of his medicine cabinet, surveying the array of 12 bottles inside. Each one represented a different attempt to manage his life. He reached for his antidepressants, which dulled his emotions but left him feeling numb. Today, he needed to be sharp and focused for a big project, so he picked out his prescription of Adderall, meant for his ADHD, and washed it down with a strong cup of coffee.

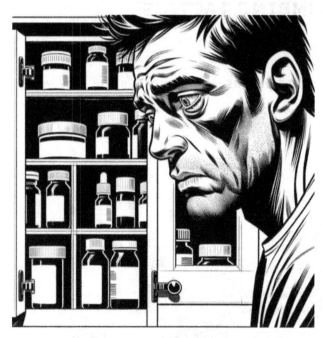

As he settled into his work, his phone pinged with an unpleasant email from a colleague. Frustrated and needing a break, Robert stepped outside for a cigarette, hoping the nicotine would calm his nerves.

Back at his desk, he grabbed a bag of potato chips and started working again, trying to drown out his stress with the crunch of snacks.

Hours passed, and when Robert finally looked down, he was surprised to see the bag of chips was empty. He couldn't even remember eating that much. Feeling queasy, he reached for a soda to settle his stomach before heading outside for another smoke. The day felt endless, and it wasn't even halfway over.

By the end of the day, exhausted from work, Robert decided to get fast food from the drive-through on his way home. Once home, he plopped down in front of the TV and flipped through the channels for a few hours, zoning out while drinking a beer. As the night drew to a close, he took an Ambien to help him fall asleep, hoping to escape the stress and fatigue of the day.

Robert's reliance on various substances to cope with his stress and emotions had become a daily routine. The antidepressants, Adderall, cigarettes, junk food, beer, and sleeping pills were all his ways of escaping reality, numbing himself to get through each day. This cycle of unhealthy numbing tactics not only affected his productivity but also took a toll on his physical and mental health.

Sedating the Soul

The knee jerk response to acute or sudden stress typically involves a physiological reaction known as the "fight or flight" response which is controlled by the sympathetic branch of our nervous system. When faced with stress, the body releases stress hormones such as adrenaline and cortisol. These hormones trigger a cascade of physiological changes designed to help the body respond to the perceived threat or challenge.

This response is often automatic and can occur even before we consciously process the stress. It's an evolutionary adaptation that helped our ancestors react quickly to danger in their environment. However, chronic or excessive stress can have negative effects on both physical and mental health over time.

When we are exposed to chronic stress, many of us turn to unhealthy coping mechanisms such as pills, food, substance use, and distraction to manage the discomfort. These behaviors may provide temporary relief, but they can ultimately worsen the stress and lead to negative health and life consequences.

Medicating Stress: A Bandage, Not a Cure

The manifestations of chronic stress are some of the top reasons many people seek medical care. Unfortunately, much of Western medicine is focused on pharmaceutical interventions to treat the symptoms rather than solving the underlying root of the problem. For example, if we are having trouble sleeping because of stress, a doctor might prescribe sleeping pills. But that does not fix what's causing the stress in the first place. It's like putting a bandage on a cut without cleaning it first.

Despite often having no lasting benefit, prescription of medications is at an all-time high. The Centers for Disease Control and Prevention (CDC) estimates the number of

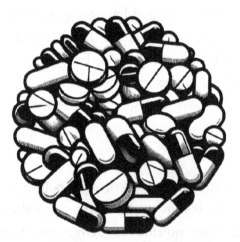

prescriptions filled in retail pharmacies was over 4.5 billion in 2019. Nearly half of all Americans used at least one prescription in the last 30 days, and almost 12% use five or more prescription drugs in that same time. The more medications we take directly increases our risk of drug interactions and adverse side effects. In general, my healthiest patients are the ones on the least amount of medications. Physicians are trying to help patients by prescribing medications, but often the side effects and interactions with other drugs simply make people worse.

Talk to a physician before stopping any medications, but in my experience, too many medications can make us sick.

The use of psychotropic medications, including antidepressants, antipsychotics, and mood stabilizers are also on the rise. Unfortunately, this has not resulted in better mental health as all of the conditions for which these medications are prescribed are skyrocketing. Over the past few decades, there has been a notable increase in the prevalence of mental illness in the United States. According to the National Institute of Mental Health (NIMH), approximately 20% of adults in the United States experience mental illness each year. The prevalence of mental

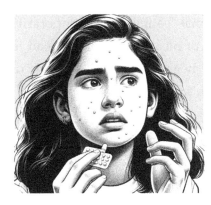

health disorders among children and adolescents has been increasing steadily. For example, the occurrence of major depressive episodes among adolescents aged 12 to 17 increased from 8.7% in 2005 to 13.3% in 2019, according to the Substance Abuse and Mental Health Services Administration (SAMHSA). Suicide rates in the United States have been rising over the past two decades. According to the CDC, the suicide rate increased by 35% from 1999 to 2018. People are more stressed and popping a pill is often not solving the problem.

Avoidance Strategies: Unhealthy Numbing Approaches

Medications are not the only unhealthy way people deal with chronic stress and anxiety. There are multiple behavioral numbing techniques and forms of distraction people use to cope.

Here are some common unhealthy ways people may deal with chronic stress:

Substance Abuse

Some individuals may turn to alcohol, drugs, or other substances as a way to numb or escape from chronic stress. While these substances may provide temporary relief, they can lead to addiction, physical health problems, and worse mental health symptoms over time.

Emotional Eating

Chronic stress can trigger cravings for comfort foods high in sugar, fat, and calories. Emotional eating may temporarily soothe stress and provide a sense of pleasure, but it can lead to weight gain, poor nutrition, and negative feelings of guilt or shame.

Avoidance and Denial

Ignoring or denying the existence of chronic stressors and the emotions they trigger in us may seem easier in the short term, but it can lead to increased anxiety, depression, and worsen stress-related symptoms in the long run. Avoidance may involve procrastination, ignoring problems, or withdrawing from social interactions.

Escapism

Engaging in excessive screen time, binge-watching TV shows or movies, or compulsively playing video games can serve as a form of escapism from chronic stress. While distraction can be beneficial in moderation, excessive escapism can lead to neglect of responsibilities, social isolation, and decreased emotional resilience.

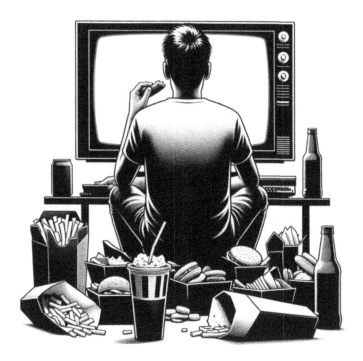

Self-Harm

In extreme cases, some individuals may resort to self-harming behaviors such as cutting, burning, or hitting themselves as a way to cope with overwhelming emotions and stress. Self-harm may provide temporary relief from emotional pain but can lead to serious physical and psychological harm.

Excessive Work

Pouring oneself into work or taking on excessive responsibilities as a way to distract from chronic stress can lead to burnout, fatigue, and strained relationships. Overworking may provide temporary relief from stress but can ultimately worsen overall well-being and satisfaction with life.

Negative Coping Patterns

Engaging in negative coping patterns such as blaming others, lashing out in anger, victimhood, or engaging in self-destructive behaviors can perpetuate a cycle of stress and dysfunction in relationships and daily life.

It is common for people to use various numbing techniques to cope with chronic stress. These behaviors can provide temporary relief from stress by distracting us and numbing our emotions. However, it is essential to recognize that relying solely on these strategies does not address the root causes of our stress and can have negative consequences on our mental and physical health down the road.

Why Do We Run Away From Our Feelings?

We need to ask ourselves do we ever use any of these numbing techniques to handle our chronic stress. This question is not

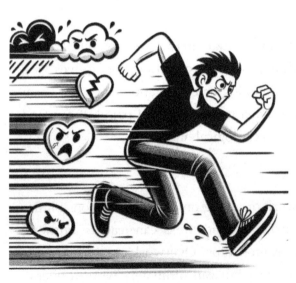

meant to make us judge ourselves or to activate that negative voice in our head that is always criticizing. That voice is not helping us. First and foremost, it is important to approach this topic without judgment or self-criticism.

We all engage in some types of avoidance strategies to some degree at different points in time. We are all doing the best we can with the tools and knowledge we have at any given moment. It is crucial to cultivate self compassion and understanding that struggling with stress is a normal part of the human experience.

As we discussed before in modern society, there is often a cultural expectation to suppress or ignore our emotions. We are taught that showing vulnerability or expressing our feelings is a sign of weakness. However, nothing could be further from the truth. Emotions are a fundamental aspect of being human, and allowing ourselves to feel them is a strength, not a weakness. In fact, embracing our emotions and being willing to experience them fully is one of the bravest things we can do. Expressing our emotions is also a way to be more authentic, deepening our connection to those around us and in influencing situations to arrive at different outcomes when done clearly and responsibly.

Being vulnerable means allowing ourselves to be open and honest about our feelings, even when it is uncomfortable or scary. It means acknowledging our pain, fear, and sadness without judgment and allowing ourselves to deal with those emotions, rather than trying to push them away or numb them.

So, are we strong enough to be vulnerable? It is a challenging question, but one worth considering. Being vulnerable requires courage and resilience. It means being willing to face our emotions head-on, even when they're painful or overwhelming. The only way out is through. In facing our emotions, we allow ourselves the opportunity to heal and grow.

Breathwork: The Transformative Alternative to Numbing

In my own experience, I have experimented with various numbing techniques to cope with chronic stress. Avoidance and distraction became my go-to methods. I would immerse myself in TV shows and social media, munching on snacks as I tried to escape from my worries. Work became my refuge, a place where I could bury myself in tasks and ignore the toll it took on my health and sleep. I bottled up my stress for so long that it would eventually erupt, affecting those around me. Despite spending over 10 years on antidepressants and undergoing talk therapy for years, that persistent feeling of stress and anxiety never seemed to go away—until I found Breathwork.

My first 90-minute session of Somatic Release Breathwork felt like five years of talk therapy. While this may not be the case for everyone, it has been the closest thing to a magic fix I've discovered. I acknowledge the valuable role of medications such as antidepressants in improving mental health—I prescribe them and have personally benefited from them. However, I also found that antidepressants left me feeling emotionally numb. Although they lifted me out of depression, they also dulled my ability to experience joy.

Similarly, talk therapy provided intellectual insight into my issues, but it didn't address the underlying root of my stress and anxiety. Despite understanding my challenges on an intellectual level, I still felt a lingering inner sense of turmoil. That's where Somatic Release and Transformational Breathwork made a profound difference. Without having to delve into traumatic memories, I was able to release pent-up emotions and traumas that had hindered my well-being for years.

I was so amazed by the transformative power of Somatic Release and Transformational Breathwork that I felt compelled to share it with others. I questioned why this effective, side-effect-free practice wasn't more widely utilized instead of medications. Breathwork is accessible to all, costs nothing, and offers lasting healing benefits. I eagerly shared this discovery with my patients, and I am thrilled to pass it on to you now.

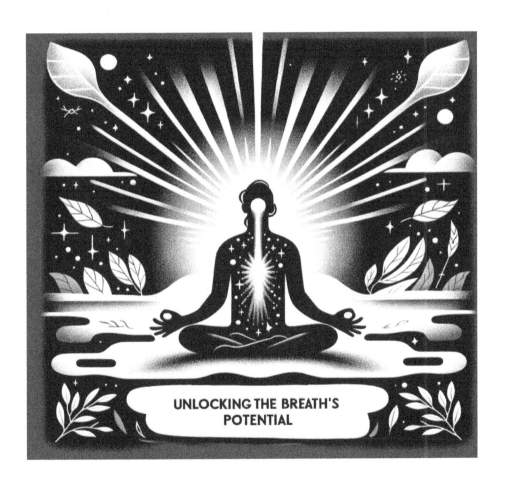

UNLOCKING THE BREATH'S POTENTIAL

4
THE SCIENCE OF BREATH

"The breath is the most vital, life-giving force in the body. Without it, we cannot exist for more than a few minutes. By mastering the breath, we can tap into its incredible potential for healing and transformation."

-Eckhart Tolle

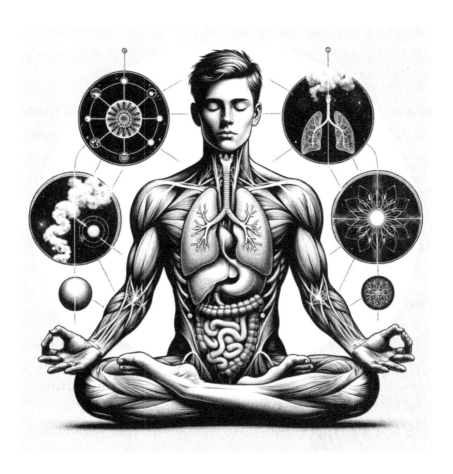

Breathing Anatomy: The Parts and Pieces

Understanding the anatomy and mechanics of breathing is essential for harnessing the power of our breath to enhance health and well-being. Gaining insight into how our breathing functions enables us to control it more adeptly, promoting relaxation and alleviating anxiety. By becoming more aware of how our breath works, we can learn to control it more effectively and use it to promote relaxation and stress relief.

Breathing marks the boundaries of our lives—from our very first breath at birth to our last at death. Despite its perpetual presence, breathing often remains unnoticed and automatic. Yet, without it, life ceases to exist. We can survive days without water and weeks without food, but a few minutes without air results in immediate peril. Breath is the vital sign of life.

Inhaling draws oxygen into our lungs, initiating its transport through our bloodstream to every cell, where it combines with glucose to generate the energy that sustains us. Breathing does much more than simply exchange gases in our lungs. It influences the pH of our blood, impacts our cardiovascular health, and even modulates our nervous system, which also affects our emotions. Let's delve into the remarkable intricacies of this life-sustaining process.

The Nose – Designed for Breathing

The respiratory system begins with the nose, a complex structure comprised of bone, cartilage, and soft tissue. Although many people tend to mouth-breathe, the mouth is actually intended for eating, speaking, and drinking. For optimal health, breathing should primarily occur through the nose—its natural purpose. We will explore specialized Breathwork techniques that involve mouth-breathing later, but generally, nasal breathing is recommended for not only the routine activities of our daily lives but also during exercise.

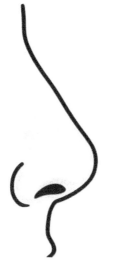

The nose features two openings, known as nostrils or nares, which lead into the nasal cavity. This cavity is lined with mucous membranes and fine, hair-like structures called cilia, which filter dust, allergens, and other airborne particles, enhancing air quality and reducing infection risk. Additionally, the nose conditions the air for the lungs by warming and humidifying it, which reduces the energy the lungs need to expend to adjust air temperature and obtain adequate moisture levels.

The Nasal Cycle

Here's a quick experiment to try: Close one nostril and feel the airflow, then switch and close the other. You'll notice that one nostril is often more open than the other, a phenomenon known as the nasal cycle. This alternation happens approximately every four hours, helping to prevent nasal dryness by distributing the workload between the nostrils. It also enhances our sense of smell, as the slower airflow in the congested nostril allows more time for scent particles to engage with our olfactory receptors. Approximately 80% of people experience this nasal cycle, illustrating its importance in our respiratory and sensory systems.

The Remarkable Role of Nitric Oxide

Nitric oxide (NO) is an extraordinary molecule produced in the nasal cavity, recognized for its pivotal roles throughout the body. In 1998, the Nobel Prize in Physiology or Medicine was awarded for the discovery of nitric oxide's crucial functions in the cardiovascular system. It acts as a potent vasodilator, relaxing and widening blood vessels, which helps regulate blood pressure and reduces the risk of blood clots. Notably, nitric oxide is a key component in medications like Viagra, enhancing blood flow to all the right places.

Beyond cardiovascular benefits, nitric oxide exhibits powerful antimicrobial properties. It can inhibit the growth of bacteria, viruses, and fungi in the nasal passages and respiratory tract, playing a significant role in defending against pathogens. Its anti-inflammatory qualities are particularly beneficial in respiratory conditions such as asthma or chronic obstructive pulmonary disease (COPD), where it helps dilate bronchi and ease airflow, reducing bronchoconstriction or narrowing of the airways. Nitric oxide assists in bronchodilation—widening the airways in the lungs, facilitating smoother airflow and enhancing oxygen uptake. More blood flow and more airflow result in better oxygenation uptake at the level of the lungs.

Moreover, nitric oxide also interacts with carbon dioxide to optimize the binding and release of oxygen from red blood cells, ensuring more efficient oxygen delivery to tissues, organs, and the brain. Nitric oxide helps oxygen to get where it needs to go.

But the benefits of nitric oxide extend even further:

- It fosters communication between nerve and brain cells, aiding memory and responsiveness.

- It reduces cholesterol levels and decreases arterial plaque, which can lead to fewer heart attacks and strokes.

- It stimulates cell growth and replication, and enhances oxygen delivery to mitochondria—the energy powerhouses of cells—boosting overall energy levels and physical performance.

- It diminishes recovery times post-exercise, reduces lactic acid buildup, and alleviates muscle soreness and fatigue.

This vital molecule is most effectively introduced into our lungs and circulated throughout our body when we breathe through our nose—not through our mouth. Mouth breathers exhibit significantly lower levels of nitric oxide. Only the nose knows NO. Thus, for the myriad benefits it offers, breathing through the nose is essential.

Interesting Fact:

Humming can increase nitric oxide production by up to 15 times. Try humming during exhales to boost heart health and maximize the many other benefits of nitric oxide.

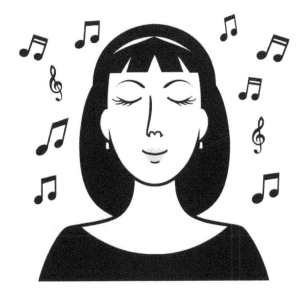

Navigating the Pharynx - A Conduit for Air and Food

The pharynx serves as a crucial passageway where both air and food travel, beginning just beyond the nasal cavity. It is structured into three distinct regions: the nasopharynx, which connects to the nasal cavity; the oropharynx, linking to the mouth; and the laryngopharynx, which leads to the larynx.

This shared pathway means that both air and food momentarily go through the same space, which can sometimes lead to complications. For instance, if food or liquid mistakenly enters the airway—a condition known as aspiration—it can cause choking or even lead to pneumonia. To prevent such incidents, it is advisable to take small bites and focus while swallowing, ensuring that food goes safely down the esophagus rather than into the air passages. After all, the lungs are designed for air, not food.

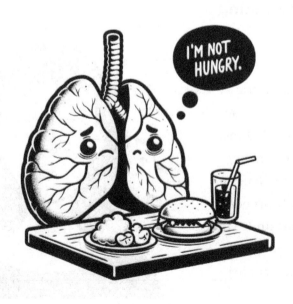

The Larynx: Gateway to Voice and Breath

Following the journey through the pharynx, air flows into the larynx, commonly referred to as the voice box. This structure houses the vocal cords and marks the entrance to the lower respiratory tract. During exhalation, the vocal cords vibrate to produce sound. Both the pitch and volume of our voice are influenced by how the vocal cords are tensed and positioned.

One notable feature of the larynx is the Adam's Apple, which is actually the protruding cartilage of the larynx. It is more prominent in males, growing significantly in response to increased testosterone levels during puberty. This structure not only contributes to the physical characteristics of the voice but also plays a pivotal role in vocal modulation and airway protection.

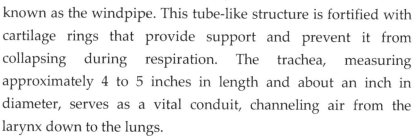

The Trachea: The Windy Windpipe

After air moves through the larynx, it enters the trachea, commonly known as the windpipe. This tube-like structure is fortified with cartilage rings that provide support and prevent it from collapsing during respiration. The trachea, measuring approximately 4 to 5 inches in length and about an inch in diameter, serves as a vital conduit, channeling air from the larynx down to the lungs.

The interior of the trachea is lined with mucous membranes and cilia—tiny hair-like structures. These cilia beat in synchronized waves, effectively moving mucus and trapped particles upwards toward the throat, where they can either be swallowed or expelled. This movement is part of the body's continuous effort to clean and moisten the air before it reaches the lungs.

Additionally, the trachea features a cough reflex, a critical protective mechanism. This reflex is triggered when the trachea's lining senses an irritant, prompting a cough to clear the airway of foreign particles, mucus, or other irritants, thus maintaining clear and safe respiratory passages.

Branching Out: The Bronchi and the Bronchial Tree

The trachea divides into two main branches, called the primary bronchi, with each one leading into a lung. These bronchi mark the beginning of what is known as the bronchial tree—a complex network of airways within the lungs. Starting with the left and right main bronchi, this branching system continues to subdivide into smaller bronchi and even finer tubes called bronchioles.

The structure of our respiratory system strikingly resembles an upside-down tree. This "tree" functions in a beautifully reciprocal relationship with actual trees: while our bronchial tree intakes oxygen and expels carbon dioxide, trees absorb carbon dioxide and release oxygen, which sustains our breathing. This fascinating symmetry highlights the interconnectedness of life and the natural world.

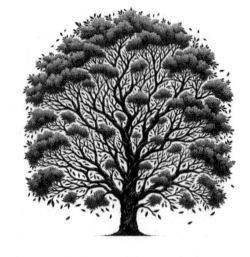

Airway Dynamics: The Role of Bronchioles

The bronchioles, smaller branches of the bronchial tree, further subdivide as the exchange occurs. These tiny airways are surrounded by smooth muscle that plays a critical role in regulating airflow. When these muscles contract, the bronchioles narrow in a process known as bronchoconstriction, which reduces airflow. Conversely, relaxation of these muscles, often stimulated by nitric oxide, causes bronchodilation, expanding the airways and increasing airflow.

In respiratory conditions such as bronchial asthma, these mechanisms can become dysfunctional. Inflammation and contraction of the smooth muscles lead to persistent bronchoconstriction, resulting in symptoms like wheezing, coughing, and shortness of breath. Understanding and managing these airway dynamics are crucial for maintaining effective breathing and managing asthma.

The Alveoli: The Convergence of Air and Blood

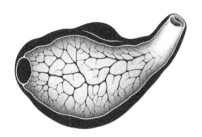

The alveoli are minuscule, balloon-like air sacs at the end of the bronchial tree within the lungs, enveloped by a dense network of capillaries. Each lung houses millions of these alveoli, creating a vast surface area—comparable to a tennis court—for the critical process of gas exchange. Here, oxygen from the inhaled air is transferred to the blood, while carbon dioxide is expelled from the blood into the lungs to be exhaled.

Air's Path in Our Lungs

To summarize the journey of air: it starts at the nose, travels through the nasal cavity, passes the pharynx, larynx, trachea, bronchi, and bronchioles, and finally arrives at the alveoli. This intricate pathway ensures that the air is effectively filtered,

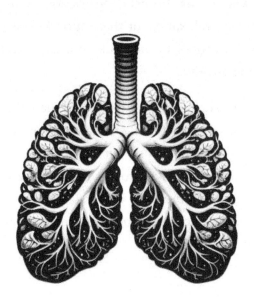

warmed, and humidified, preparing it for the most efficient gas exchange at the alveolar level. This intricate system underscores the sophisticated design of the respiratory tract, optimized to support essential life functions.

Breathing Dynamics: A Deep Dive into Respiratory Mechanics

Understanding the mechanics of breathing requires exploring how gases and pressure interact. Gases naturally move from areas of high pressure to areas of low pressure, seeking spaces where they are less compressed.

To make it simple, we can understand breathing as governed by two main pressures: atmospheric pressure, which is the external air pressure typically at 760 mmHg, and intrapulmonary pressure, which is the pressure within the lungs.

Intrapulmonary pressure fluctuates slightly around atmospheric pressure during breathing, decreasing during inhalation and increasing during exhalation because of changes in lung volume.

These changes in lung volume are facilitated by the contraction and relaxation of respiratory muscles, primarily the diaphragm and intercostal muscles, as well as additional muscles in the chest, neck, and abdomen. Together, these muscles expand and contract the thoracic chest cavity, allowing air to flow in and out of the lungs.

Most of us know about the diaphragm and that it has something to do with breathing, but what does it look like? It turns out the diaphragm looks like a dome underneath our lungs. When it contracts on inhalation, it actually moves downward and flattens, pulling the lungs downward which increase their volume. The increased volume means less pressure inside than outside so the air flows in. This might seem counterintuitive, as "contraction" typically implies a decrease in size, but the unique shape and function of the diaphragm explain this phenomenon. Similarly, the intercostal muscles, situated between the ribs, assist in lifting and expanding the rib cage during inhalation, further increasing thoracic chest volume.

Exhalation, or expiration, is the process of letting air out of the lungs during the respiratory cycle. When the breathing muscles relax and the lung tissue elastically recoils, lung volume decreases. Decreased volume means the pressure inside the lungs goes up and forces air out of the lungs, because air wants to move toward the area of lower pressure outside.

Together, these processes of inhalation and exhalation constitute the fundamental actions of breathing, showcasing the dynamic and sophisticated nature of our respiratory system.

Why Do We Breathe?

At first glance, the question "Why do we breathe?" might seem silly. Obviously, we breathe to live—and because we do not like the alternative. We have to breathe to survive. Yet, the fundamental reason we breathe goes beyond mere survival; it's about energy—the very essence of life.

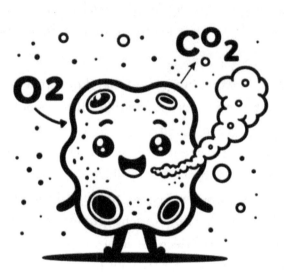

Breathing powers cellular respiration, a complex biochemical process that fuels every action and reaction in our bodies. Through inhalation, we intake oxygen, which is then transported from our lungs to every tissue and cell via the bloodstream. This oxygen is crucial for the metabolic processes that occur in the mitochondria, the little energy factories of our cells.

Here's how it works: oxygen, carried by red blood cells, reaches every part of our body. The exchange of oxygen from the red blood cells to the cells of tissues and organs is a finely tuned process that can be modified by how much carbon dioxide and nitric oxide are in the blood. The exchange from the blood to the tissue cells is crucial for our body's function. Once inside a cell, oxygen is used by the mitochondria in conjunction with glucose—the primary energy source derived from our food. The result of this reaction is adenosine triphosphate (ATP), the energy currency of the cell, along with the byproducts of water and carbon dioxide.

The chemical equation can be summarized as:

Oxygen + Glucose → ATP (energy) + Water + Carbon Dioxide

In essence, every breath we take converts to energy via a magnificent series of biochemical reactions, highlighting how integral breathing is not just for survival, but for sustaining every function within our body. Thus, breath is not merely air; it's one of our primary sources of energy, making it a fundamental aspect of life itself.

The Air We Share: Breaking Down What We Breathe

The air around us is a mixture predominantly composed of nitrogen and oxygen, along with smaller amounts of other gases. When we inhale, about 78% of the air is nitrogen, 21% is oxygen, and a minor 0.04% is carbon

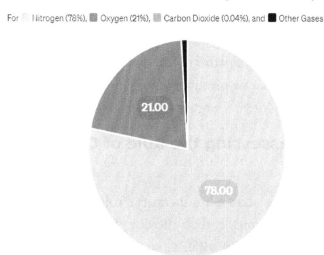

For ⬜ Nitrogen (78%), ⬛ Oxygen (21%), ⬜ Carbon Dioxide (0.04%), and ⬛ Other Gases

dioxide, with trace amounts of other gases like argon and helium.

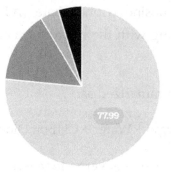

Nitrogen (77.99%), ■ Oxygen (15%), ■ Carbon Dioxide (4%), ■ Water Vapor (5%), and Other Gases

Upon exhaling, the composition of the air we breathe out changes due to the biochemical processes that occur within our bodies. The exhaled air contains approximately 77.999% nitrogen—a very slight decrease from what we inhaled. The oxygen content drops to about 15%, reflecting the oxygen that has been used in metabolic processes to produce energy. Notably, the carbon dioxide content increases significantly, up to about 4%, as a byproduct of cellular respiration. Additionally, our exhaled breath includes roughly 5% water vapor, a result of the humidifying process that air undergoes in the respiratory system and the moisture produced in cellular respiration. This shift in gas percentages between inhaled and exhaled air underscores the body's efficient use of oxygen and its role in expelling carbon dioxide, which is crucial for maintaining a balanced internal environment. Furthermore, this delicate balance is essential for cellular respiration, energy production, and the overall functioning of vital organs.

Oxygen's Ally: Reassessing the Role of Carbon Dioxide

While oxygen often receives acclaim for its crucial role in fueling the body's biochemical reactions, carbon dioxide (CO_2), its less celebrated counterpart, is equally vital. Commonly labeled as merely a "waste gas", this view overlooks carbon dioxide's essential functions. CO_2 not only assists oxygen in detaching from red blood cells to nourish body tissues but also plays a significant role in dilating the body's extensive network of blood vessels, maintaining acid-base balance, and facilitating waste elimination.

Air Hunger

Let's explore the body's breathing impulse with a simple experiment: Take a deep breath in, exhale completely, and then hold your breath. How long is it before you feel the urge to breathe again? This 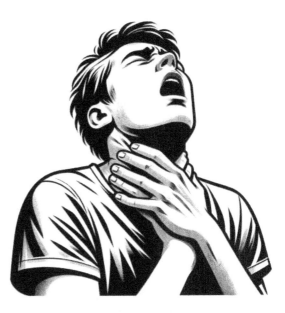 sensation is called "air hunger" and is the intense, uncomfortable strong urge to breathe more deeply or rapidly. What is driving this urge? Most people think it is a lack of oxygen. Wrong. It is actually an increase in CO_2 levels.

Despite common beliefs, oxygen levels in healthy adults remain steady (between 95% and 100%) regardless of breathing pace. Taking deeper or more frequent breaths doesn't "top off" our oxygen levels since our blood typically carries a full load of oxygen. The compelling need to breathe comes not from a lack of oxygen, but from an increase in CO_2 levels.

To see this in action, repeat the breath-holding exercise and monitor your oxygen levels with a pulse oximeter. You'll notice the sensation of needing to breathe or air hunger arises well before any significant drop in oxygen saturation. This urge usually kicks in after just 10 to 40 seconds of breath-holding, though it can take up to three minutes of holding your breath to see a noticeable decrease in oxygen saturation.

This air hunger is because of rising CO_2 levels. Our bodies have specialized chemoreceptors that monitor these levels in our bloodstream. When CO_2 accumulates, these receptors stimulate the brainstem's respiratory centers to increase the rate and depth of breathing. Thus, in healthy individuals, the primary driver for breathing is not the need for more oxygen, but the regulation of carbon dioxide levels, highlighting its underestimated yet critical role in our respiratory system.

Chronic Stress Triggers Habitual Overbreathing

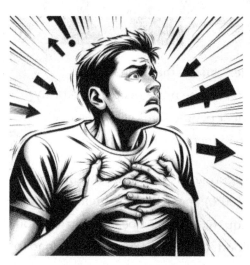

The role of CO_2 as a primary trigger for breathing introduces a critical issue in modern life: chronic overbreathing linked to heightened stress responses. Our sympathetic nervous system activates the "fight or flight" response which is appropriate when fleeing danger like an angry bear but problematic when it becomes a chronic reaction to everyday stressors. This leads to increased respiration, which, over time, can recalibrate the body's CO_2 chemoreceptors to a lower sensitivity, causing rapid-shallow-chest breathing even when it is unnecessary.

Rapid-shallow-chest breathing tells our heart to tell our brain that we are in danger which perpetuates the fast breathing. This dysfunctional cycle can perpetuate chronic stress and anxiety.

In today's fast-paced world, many of us breathe too quickly as a result of constant stress from factors like processed foods, lack of exercise, technology overload, and poor sleep. This habitual stress breathing affects an estimated 50% to 60% of people, keeping their bodies in a perpetual state of alert. Fast, shallow breathing not only maintains high stress levels but also reduces CO_2 levels as we breathe out more CO_2. This leads to constricted blood vessels and less oxygen able to release from our red blood cells which decreases oxygen reaching vital organs, including the brain and heart. This can cause mental fog and reduced body efficiency.

Chronic stress not only recalibrates our body's sensitivity to carbon dioxide, leading to rapid-shallow-chest breathing, but also affects our breathing habits in noticeable ways. We sigh more frequently when we are frustrated or under chronic stress, which is a reflex to release excess carbon dioxide as a result of our lower threshold because of chronic overbreathing. During periods of stress, we may also find ourselves breathing audibly and primarily through our mouths. Interestingly, some people respond to stress by holding their breath, which is often followed by frequent sighing to compensate for the build-up of carbon dioxide.

This altered breathing behavior, whether it's overbreathing, mouth breathing, or frequent sighing keeps our bodies in a heightened state of alertness and contributes to a cycle of continuous stress. By engaging in these patterns, we inadvertently reinforce the body's stress response, impacting our overall health and well-being. A chronically elevated heart rate is a tell-tale sign we may be overbreathing.

Moreover, overbreathing leads to a significant reduction in carbon dioxide levels within the body, which causes blood vessels to constrict. This reduction in blood vessel diameter can impede the flow of blood and reduce the oxygen supply to various parts of the body. A common symptom of this is having cold hands and feet, which is a possible indicator of chronic overbreathing.

The Paradox of Slowing Down: More Oxygen, Less Stress

Counterintuitively, slowing down our breathing can actually enhance oxygen delivery throughout the body. Remember our friend nitric oxide? It works alongside CO2 to facilitate the

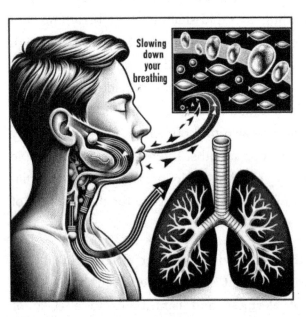

transfer of oxygen from red blood cells to tissues. Rapid, mouth-based breathing depletes CO2 and bypasses nitric oxide production in the nose, impairing this process. By slowing our breath or even holding it briefly, we increase CO2, which can initially trigger air hunger, but remember there is no need to panic—our oxygen levels are stable. Letting the CO_2 level rise dilates blood vessels and facilitates oxygen leaving red blood cells and going into the tissue which improves blood and oxygen flow to the brain and other organs, and ultimately enhances overall circulation.

Even if we are breathing through our nose, if we are still overbreathing, the carbon dioxide in our blood is lower than needed for optimal oxygen transfer. One of the biggest things we can do to decrease our feeling of stress is to reset our carbon dioxide threshold for air hunger and breathe lower and slower.

Practical Experiment: Realigning Our Breath

Try this simple test: Place one hand on your chest and one on your belly, and take a deep breath. Did your chest or belly rise first? Most often, stress induces chest breathing, which perpetuates anxiety. The common advice to "take a deep breath" can backfire if done incorrectly when we take a big gulp of air through our mouth into our chest. Instead, breathe slowly and deeply into the diaphragm through the nose to truly lessen stress.

Continuous overbreathing can lead to significant reductions in brain oxygenation—up to 50%—impairing cognitive function. Slower breathing not only helps us think clearer but is also essential in managing chronic anxiety. Studies, such as those conducted at the University of Albany, show that individuals with high anxiety typically breathe faster and have lower CO_2 levels, which can worsen their anxiety in a cyclical feedback loop. It becomes a "which came first: the chicken or the egg" scenario. People breathe faster when they are anxious but then breathing faster causes anxiety. These negative feedback loops underline the importance of conscious intervention in our unconscious cycles. Breathe slower to think better.

Understanding the dual roles of oxygen and CO2 in our respiratory system challenges us to reconsider the importance of balanced breathing. By adopting slower, more mindful breathing techniques, we can disrupt the cycles of stress and anxiety, improving our mental clarity and physiological health. This conscious intervention transforms our approach to stress and the very air we breathe.

Establishing Your Baseline: The Breath Hold Time Test

Understanding our baseline carbon dioxide tolerance is crucial for gauging our respiratory health and measuring improvement over time. A simple yet effective way to assess this is through the Breath Hold Time (BHT) test. Despite being commonly referred to in medical contexts as the Body Oxygen Level Test (the BOLT score), calling it the Breath Hold Time or BHT is more accurately focused on carbon dioxide tolerance rather than oxygen levels, which typically remain stable.

The BHT measures how long we can comfortably hold our breath before the onset of air hunger which is a direct indicator of our body's tolerance to carbon dioxide and reflects the efficiency of our breathing patterns. As such, BHT serves as a valuable self-assessment tool to monitor respiratory health and the effectiveness of breathing retraining techniques.

Over time, tracking changes in the BHT score can provide insights into improvements in our breathing patterns and overall respiratory function. It is a straightforward method that requires nothing more than our breath and a stopwatch, making it accessible for regular self-monitoring.

Variations in BHT scores can depend on several factors including age, fitness level, respiratory health, and lifestyle habits. Individuals who frequently experience overbreathing typically have shorter BHT scores. Research has linked low BHT scores with various respiratory conditions, such as asthma, chronic obstructive pulmonary disease (COPD), and anxiety-related breathing disorders. Consequently, improving our BHT through targeted breathing retraining can significantly enhance respiratory health and reduce symptoms associated with these conditions.

It's important to note that the BHT is not about pushing ourselves to the limit, as we might have done as children during breath-holding contests. Instead, this test focuses on the moment air hunger first begins—not the maximum duration we can forcibly hold our breath. This approach avoids the influence of factors that can be consciously controlled and provides a more accurate

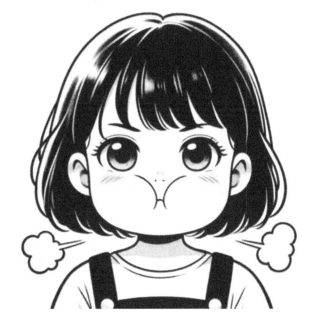

assessment of our natural respiratory responses and carbon dioxide sensitivity. This will give us a meaningful measure of our current baseline for carbon dioxide tolerance and help guide effective interventions for better respiratory health.

Setting Your BHT Benchmark

Find a comfortable sitting position and relax. Prepare a timing device that counts seconds—your phone's stopwatch will suffice. Begin by taking a normal breath in, then exhale fully. Pinch your nose to seal off any air entry. Watch the timer and note how many seconds pass until you experience the initial desire to breathe. Remember, this exercise is not about testing your limits; if you find yourself gasping for air when you release your nose, you've extended too far, and the measurement won't reflect your true Breath Hold Time (BHT).

A BHT of 40 seconds is often indicative of a healthy and fit body, but it's rare for even professional athletes to achieve this

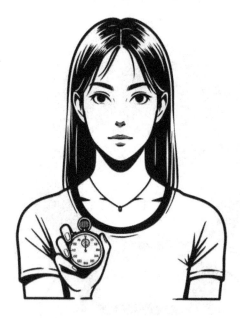

on their first try. Many people start with a BHT of only 10 to 15 seconds— mine was 12 seconds. However, the good news is that improving your CO_2 tolerance—and thereby increasing your BHT—is entirely manageable through practice and breathing exercises.

For the most accurate measurement, perform this test right after waking up. Morning values tend to be the lowest of the day but are the most reflective of our natural respiratory baseline. This initial score is our starting point, and regular monitoring can help us observe improvements over time as we engage in breathing retraining practices.

Enhancing Our CO2 Tolerance is Key to Chronic Stress Relief

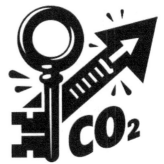

Improving our carbon dioxide tolerance is a crucial strategy for managing chronic stress and fostering healthier breathing patterns for everyday life. By addressing overbreathing, we send a calming signal to our heart that all is well, which in turn communicates to the brain to relax. This foundational shift not only helps us approach life's challenges from a place of calm but also enhances oxygen delivery to our brain, improving our overall resilience and cognitive function.

The goal is to fundamentally change how we breathe into a low and slow rhythm. We aim to bring air deep into our abdomen by engaging our diaphragm and slowing our respiratory rate. Initially, we have to consciously focus on breathing the right way, and it's natural to often forget as our attention is pulled in many directions. When we do remember, we simply start again.

This learning process follows a progression: we begin with unconscious incompetence, where we are unaware of our ineffective breathing habits. Then we move to conscious incompetence, where we recognize the problem but may struggle to change it. Next, we reach conscious competence, where we can breathe correctly with effort. Finally, we achieve unconscious competence, where effective breathing becomes second nature. By committing to this practice, we can transform our breath and, consequently, our overall well-being.

Techniques for Increasing CO2 Tolerance

Several practical techniques can help increase our CO2 tolerance. A simple method is to see how many paces you can walk while holding your breath. Another effective technique is the Breathe Light to Breathe Right method, popularized by Patrick McKeown, author of *The Oxygen Advantage* and *The Breathing Cure*. This method involves deliberately reducing our breath volume to create a manageable level of air hunger, which helps reset the brain's CO2 tolerance threshold, leading to naturally slower and more efficient breathing. For more structured approaches, resources like TheBreathMD.com offer guidance.

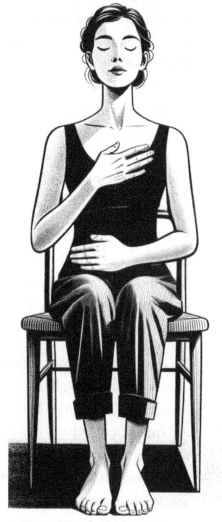

Breathe Light to Breathe Right: A Method by Patrick McKeown

Begin by sitting upright with your spine straight, allowing your shoulders to relax. Place one hand on your chest and the other on your abdomen. As you inhale, feel your belly expand gently; as you exhale, feel it contract. Apply gentle pressure with your hands to provide slight resistance to your breathing, which helps in controlling the breath's volume.

Focus on reducing the size of each breath. Inhale less air than usual, making each breath smaller and shorter. Allow each exhale to be relaxed and natural. Gradually slow down your breathing movements until you experience a manageable level of air hunger—this sensation should be noticeable but not overwhelming.

If you notice any tensing, jerking of stomach muscles, or if your breathing feels disrupted or uncontrolled, the intensity of air shortage might be too high. If this occurs, pause the exercise for about 15 seconds and resume once you feel more comfortable. Initially, you may only sustain this mild air shortage for about 20 seconds, but with practice, you can extend this period.

The aim is to maintain this rotation of manageable air hunger for three to five minutes at a time. Completing two sets of this five-minute exercise daily can effectively reset our breathing center and enhance our body's CO_2 tolerance.

Practicing this exercise increases the CO_2 levels in our blood, leading to noticeable physical changes such as a warm sensation from dilated blood vessels, a rosy complexion, and an increase in saliva production. These signs indicate we are doing it correctly, and our body is entering a state of relaxation and activating the parasympathetic nervous system, fostering a deep sense of calm throughout our system.

By engaging in this practice, we transition from a chronic sympathetic fight or flight state to a place of calm, which is fundamental to combating our chronic stress. Just 3 to 5 minutes of slowing down the breath can shift the body from the sympathetic to a parasympathetic state, providing a powerful tool for stress management. This method is also effective for relieving headaches. Give it a try and experience the benefits.

Why Mouth Breathing at Night is Harmful

Breathing through the mouth during nighttime can undermine even the best daytime breathing practices. It has several detrimental effects on health, ranging from impacting sleep quality to promoting poor oral health.

Mouth breathing at night can dry out the mouth, leading to a decrease in saliva production which is essential for neutralizing oral bacteria and acids. This condition significantly increases the risk of dental decay and gum disease. Moreover, it can worsen or lead to snoring and obstructive sleep apnea—a condition that not only disrupts sleep but is also associated with serious long-term health issues like cardiovascular disease.

For children, habitual mouth breathing can alter facial development, potentially resulting in elongated facial structures and dental malocclusions. Additionally, nighttime mouth breathing can cause frequent awakenings to urinate, as it disrupts the body's natural balance and sleep cycles.

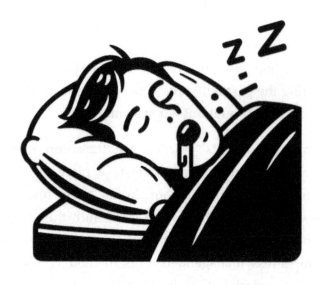

Identifying Nighttime Mouth Breathing

How can you tell if you are breathing through your mouth at night? Common indicators include waking up with a dry mouth or sore throat, snoring, and feeling fatigued despite getting a full night's sleep. If you find yourself getting up multiple times during the night to urinate, this too could be a sign of mouth breathing. Your sleeping partner might also notice these symptoms, particularly snoring.

Sleep Tape: A Simple Solution to Nighttime Mouth Breathing

The only way to be sure you don't breathe through your mouth at night is to tape it shut. Sleep taping at night often evokes a mixture of curiosity and concern when mentioned, but it's far from being a form of torture or an odd kink. It's a straightforward technique aimed at ensuring you breathe through your nose rather than your mouth while sleeping.

Although taping the mouth closed with one horizontal strip of tape is an option—it really doesn't matter what pattern is used as long as the mouth stays closed—the usual method involves placing a small, one-inch strip of surgical tape vertically from the top lip to the 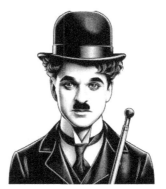 bottom, resembling a 'Charlie Chaplain mustache' positioned just over the lips. This setup is effective even for those with facial hair and is designed to keep the mouth closed while still allowing enough space at the mouth's corners for coughing, sneezing, or even mumbling a sleepy word or two to your partner.

If you are exploring a sleep taping method, you might consider using specialty tapes designed for nighttime mouth closure, although economical alternatives such as surgical tape found at any drug store work well too. I personally use one piece of painter's tape horizontally and another piece stretched from above my upper lip to under my chin, which also helps keep my

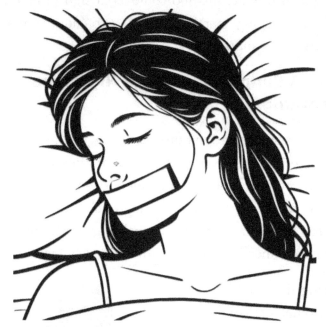

jaw closed — no more waking up to a drool-soaked pillow!

Initially, adapting to sleep tape can be challenging. It wasn't uncommon for me to find the tape removed and lying beside me during the early nights. However, by the third night, I was able to sleep through without removing the tape. In fact, I eventually found putting the tape on my mouth signaled to my brain it was time to go to sleep, and I fell asleep faster. The benefits were clear and quick: my chronic sinusitis and its associated congestion improved dramatically within a week. I noticed a reduction in nighttime bathroom trips—from three or four times a night to just once, at most. The overall quality of my sleep improved significantly, leading to deeper sleep and fewer awakenings. Over time, this led to increased daytime energy and less overall fatigue.

After about three months of consistent use, my nighttime mouth breathing habit was largely corrected. Now, if I experience a relapse during a cold or similar illness that forces me to mouth breathe, causing me to wake up with a dry mouth and a damp pillow, I return to sleep taping briefly to reinstate the habit of nasal breathing.

While the idea of sleep taping might sound unconventional at first, it has been a game-changer for many, including myself. It's a simple, yet effective way to improve sleep quality and address issues related to mouth breathing. If you're seeking a better night's sleep and the myriad health benefits that come with proper breathing, sleep taping is definitely worth considering.

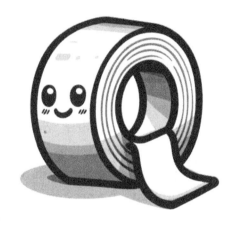

Harnessing the Power of Breath

Throughout this chapter, we have explored the intricate anatomy and profound functions of the respiratory system, from the initial intake of air through the nose, enriched by nitric oxide, down to the critical exchange in the alveoli where oxygen meets blood. We have explored how breathing is not just a biological necessity, but a powerful influence to our overall health, capable of shaping a response to stress, impacting our sleep quality, and determining our energy levels.

Through a detailed examination of the mechanics and dynamics of breathing, we have seen how the simple act of inhaling and exhaling involves a sophisticated interplay of anatomical structures and biochemical reactions. We've uncovered the often overlooked importance of carbon dioxide and addressed the modern challenge of chronic stress and its effect on our breathing patterns.

Practical strategies, such as the "Breathe Light to Breathe Right" technique, offer methods to improve our respiratory health and, by extension, our life quality. The discussion on sleep taping illuminated a simple yet effective way to ensure nasal breathing at night, highlighting the tangible benefits of such practices.

As we close this chapter, remember that each breath is a testament to life's miraculous complexity. By understanding and respecting the science of breath, we empower ourselves to live more healthfully, harnessing the power of each inhale and exhale to its fullest potential. By mastering the art of breathing, we can transform an automatic function into a tool for enhancing well-being and vitality. Let's continue to breathe well, live well, and thrive.

5
THE MIND, BODY, AND BREATH CONNECTION

"Breath is the bridge which connects life to consciousness, which unites your body to your thoughts."

- Thich Nhat Hanh

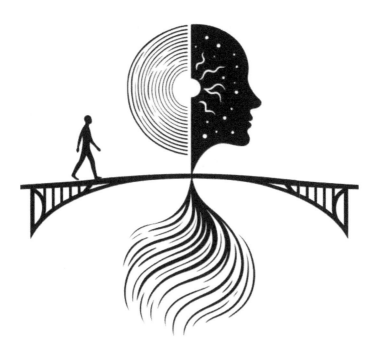

Integrating Mind-Body-Breath

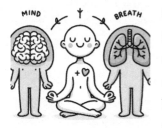

Our mind, body, and breath are all interconnected—what affects one affects the other. By nurturing these elements and their connection, we can enhance our overall well-being, fostering a balanced state that promotes mental clarity, physical health, and emotional stability. This connection between mind, body, and breath is the key to understanding how Breathwork can help us manage stress and promote overall well-being.

Breath: The Language Between the Mind and Body

Breath is like the silent conductor of the symphony between our minds and our bodies. It serves as a bridge connecting the two. The breath is not just about getting oxygen; it's about how our breath affects how we feel in our bodies. In countless cultures and spiritual traditions, the act of conscious breathing is revered as a powerful tool for achieving harmony, balance, and well-being. This ancient wisdom finds residence in modern scientific research, which increasingly recognizes the profound influence of breath on both mental and physical health.

At its core, the breath embodies the fundamental connection between the mind and the body. When we are stressed, anxious or scared, the breath serves as a mirror, reflecting our inner state and emotional landscape by becoming shallow and rapid like when we are running away from something. The breath mirrors the activation of our "fight or flight" response. Conversely, during moments of calm, relaxation, and meditation, our breath becomes slow, deep, and rhythmic, signaling the activation of our "rest and digest" response.

Breath serves as the language that speaks fluently to both the mind and the body. By cultivating awareness of our breath and harnessing its transformative power, we can cultivate resilience, balance, and wholeness in our lives. We can learn to speak the language of our body and mind, helping us feel better and live happier.

The Brain as Boss

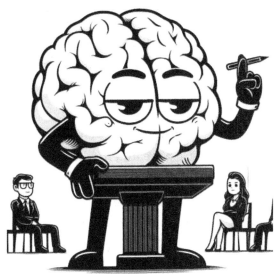

In the past, the medical community thought the brain was in charge, like a boss giving orders to the body. It was believed the brain controlled everything and the body was simply there to carry it around. However, it is not that simple. Rather, a sophisticated communication network exists, facilitating bidirectional information flow between the brain and various bodily organs. There is an exchange system in our bodies where the brain and other organs communicate back and forth. Our brain needs our body and our body needs our brain.

That said, our brains are truly remarkable and have abilities we often don't fully appreciate. They do more than just think and react; they help us understand the world, connect with others, and even heal. Our brain works with the rest of our body to keep us healthy, adapt to challenges, and recover from illnesses. This intricate system highlights how interconnected and dependent on each other every part of our body truly is.

The Placebo Effect

During my time in medical school, we didn't focus much on the idea that our thoughts could significantly affect our physical health. We were aware of the placebo effect, but most of us dismissed it as patients merely fooling themselves, rather than understanding the deep connection between the mind and the body.

The placebo effect is a fascinating phenomenon that highlights the intricate relationship between the cognitive and the physical. It refers to the mental and physical changes a person experiences when receiving a treatment like a sugar pill simply because the individual believes it will work. Essentially, the placebo effect demonstrates the power of expectation and perception in 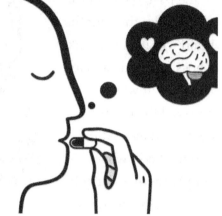 influencing our health and well-being. The placebo effect shows how much our thoughts and beliefs can affect how we feel in our bodies.

Placebos are pretty amazing. They appear to provide relief from nearly every symptom imaginable, benefiting at least 30% of patients and sometimes as many as 60%. At the heart of the placebo effect is the profound influence of the mind on the body. When we believe our treatment will alleviate our symptoms or improve our condition, our brain releases neurotransmitters and endorphins, which can lead to actual physiological changes. These changes can manifest as pain relief, reduced anxiety, improved mood, or even enhanced immune function, despite the absence of any active medical intervention.

In research settings, placebo-controlled trials are often conducted to evaluate the efficacy of new drugs or treatments. Participants are randomly assigned to receive either the active treatment or a placebo, allowing researchers to isolate the specific effects of the treatment from those resulting from the participants' expectations. Remarkably, even when individuals receive a placebo, they may experience significant improvements in their symptoms, sometimes to a degree comparable to those receiving the actual treatment. Even though the placebo treatment is not supposed to do anything, many people still feel better after taking it simply because they believed it would help.

The placebo effect underscores the importance of understanding the mind-body connection in health and disease. If our mind and thoughts can make us feel better, it only makes sense that our mind and thoughts can also make us feel worse. The placebo effect teaches us that sometimes, just believing in something can make a real difference in how we feel. What we think and believe can affect our health and well-being. The mind is a powerful thing.

States of Awareness: The Unconscious and Subconscious Mind

As we delve deeper into the mind–body–breath connection, we need to investigate the psychological framework of the mind starting with states of awareness. Within the human mind there are different levels of awareness with the most obvious being conscious versus non-conscious. Conscious is the part of the mind that you are aware of. You can verbalize about your conscious experience and you can think about it in a logical function. Non-conscious describes mental processing that occurs outside of conscious awareness. I choose to use the term "non-conscious" to describe what is outside our state of awareness rather than "unconscious" because of the frequently confusing terms used in psychology as described below.

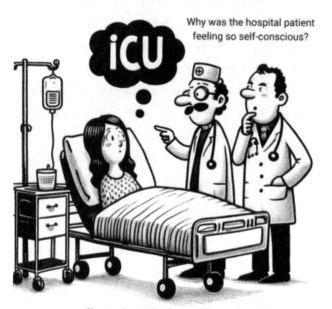

Why was the hospital patient feeling so self-conscious?

She overheard the doctors keep saying ICU

Although the terms "unconscious" and "subconscious" are frequently interchanged, the subconscious plays an important and specific role within the level of awareness of which we are not conscious. While both terms refer to aspects of mental activity that occur outside of conscious awareness (in the non-conscious), the subconscious is often seen as a level just beneath consciousness, influencing everyday thoughts and behaviors, whereas the unconscious is considered a deeper, more hidden realm of the mind containing repressed memories and powerful psychological forces. These terms have frequently frustrated me as it seems what is "not conscious" is "unconscious," but psychology has broken the realm of the non-conscious into "subconscious" (meaning "just below the conscious") and "unconscious" (literally meaning "not conscious" but used to mean "really extremely not conscious").

The subconscious is the part of our non-conscious mind responsible for processing information and experiences that are below the level of conscious awareness but can still influence thoughts, feelings, and behavior. The subconscious mind encompasses various automatic or semiautomatic processes, such as habits, learned skills, automatic reactions, hardwired beliefs and perceptions, and unconscious biases. Subconscious processes, while not in the forefront of the mind, can be brought into consciousness more easily and are often parts of our cognition that we can access with some focus or prompting. It is like a recording device as it records and logs everything you have ever experienced. It is performing millions of processes all at once. It is like the background of the mind, influencing our conscious experiences without our direct awareness of it. It is said that it is 1 million times more powerful than your conscious mind. The patterns often set in childhood are still running the show.

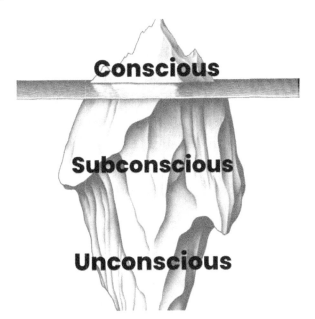

The unconscious is the part of our minds that holds information and processes at a deeper level of mental activity that is inaccessible to conscious awareness. Unconscious processes are completely unreachable to the conscious mind and affect behavior without our thinking mind being aware. We cannot access the deep unconscious level of awareness from our everyday conscious state. Examples of the unconscious include repressed memories of child abuse, unresolved conflicts, thoughts or beliefs we are not consciously aware of, repressed feelings (with more description of the difference between repression and suppression to come), and primitive instincts. According to Freud, the unconscious mind contains thoughts, feelings, desires, and memories that are too threatening or painful to be brought into conscious awareness.

The iceberg is often used to help explain these concepts. The tip of the iceberg is what you can see and represents our conscious awareness in this analogy. The unconscious can be compared to the deep, hidden base of the iceberg submerged well below the water surface. This part is vast and inaccessible, containing all the deep-seated desires, fears, and motivations that are completely removed from our conscious awareness. The subconscious, on the other hand, is like the part of the iceberg that is just below the water surface. While it is not immediately visible or actively thought about, it can be accessed more easily than the deep unconscious. The subconscious includes information that you can pull into your conscious mind when needed, like memories or learned skills that can come to the surface with a little effort or in response to a trigger.

Connor's Story: The Scarcity Mindset

Connor was a little boy in the second grade, and his class had a special contest that year. The students earned tickets for good behavior, extra credit assignments, and going above and beyond in their schoolwork. Connor was determined to earn as many tickets as possible. He worked hard all year, dreaming of one thing: a bouncy ball that lit up when it hit the ground. He talked about it constantly to his parents, describing how much he wanted it and even dreaming about playing with it.

Finally, the day of the auction arrived. The classroom buzzed with excitement as the children gathered to bid on various items with their hard-earned tickets. The first item up for auction was a kazoo, but Connor wasn't interested, so he didn't bid. Next came a charm bracelet, but that didn't catch his eye either. Then, at last, the bouncy ball came up. Connor's heart raced. He knew this was his moment.

To his dismay, many of his classmates also wanted the bouncy ball. A fierce bidding war ensued, with the price of the bouncy ball climbing higher and higher. Fortunately, Connor had worked so hard all year that he had more tickets than anyone else. He kept bidding, determined not to let his dream slip away. Finally, he won the bouncy ball! He was ecstatic, holding his prize tightly, the glow from the ball reflecting the joy in his eyes.

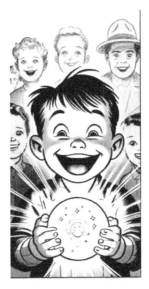

After the bouncy ball was sold, the auction continued with multiple more items. By this time, most of the children had run out of tickets, having bid on the earlier items. Only two little girls in the class had any tickets left. They had saved their tickets and were now able to buy all the remaining items at very low costs.

When the auction ended, the teacher took the opportunity to teach a lesson about saving. She praised the two little girls for their restraint and foresight, explaining that by saving their tickets, they could buy more items. Connor, who had been so happy with his bouncy ball, suddenly felt a wave of shame. The teacher's words made him feel like he had made a mistake by spending all his tickets on one item, even though it was exactly what he wanted.

This idea planted itself deeply in Connor's mind, influencing him throughout his life. Despite growing up in a household where he was never deprived of anything, he developed a scarcity mindset. He felt ashamed to spend his money, always fearing that if he did, he wouldn't have enough. This belief led him to deprive himself of things he wanted, constantly saving instead of enjoying the fruits of his labor.

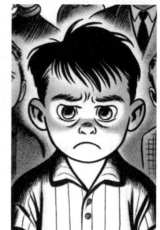

Connor's story illustrates how a single experience in childhood can shape our beliefs and behaviors for years to come. The lesson he learned that day in second grade became a subconscious rule that guided his financial decisions, leaving him with a sense of scarcity despite living a life of plenty.

Repression Versus Suppression

Repression and suppression are both psychological defense mechanisms to cope with uncomfortable or distressing thoughts, emotions, or memories. We all have trapped emotions accumulated from every moment in our life that we denied ourselves the feeling part of any intense experience. Sometimes we are aware of these emotions but other times we are not.

Repression refers to the unconscious process of our brain blocking or burying distressing thoughts, emotions, or memories from awareness. We do not even realize they are there. Repression is an unconscious process which is not voluntary. This protects us from the emotional pain associated with the experience. An example of repression is a woman who suffered sexual abuse as a child but has no active memory of it. It is very hard to work on things when we are not even aware of them.

Suppression, on the other hand, refers to the conscious process of intentionally pushing unwanted thoughts, feelings, and memories out of awareness. Suppression is a conscious process which is voluntary. This is done by actively trying to not think about or focus on the unpleasant emotions by actively choosing not to think about or acknowledge these distressing experiences. Suppressed memories and emotions are still accessible but we are most of the time pushing them out of our awareness. For example, you are at work and it would be socially unacceptable to cry so you hold it in. This is an example of suppression.

Repression and suppression lead to significant challenges, as they involve emotions that are unresolved, necessitating eventual confrontation and resolution. Over time, these trapped emotions can contribute to psychological distress or manifest as physical symptoms, making it crucial to address them for overall well-being.

The Non-Conscious is Running the Show

It is often suggested that up to 95% of our behavior and decision-making is directed by the content of our non-conscious mind, which is executed by our subconscious. Consider the common experience of driving to a destination and then realizing upon arrival that you have no memory of the journey. This phenomenon illustrates how much of our daily activity operates outside of our conscious awareness—on autopilot, so to speak.

Research indicates that humans have between 60,000 to 70,000 thoughts per day. Of these thoughts, studies suggest that 70% to 80% are negative, disempowering, self-sabotaging, and limiting. Furthermore, 95% of these negative thoughts are repetitive, cycling through our minds on a continuous loop. This pattern suggests that we are not as consciously in control of our lives as we might believe.

Instead, we are largely governed by non-conscious patterns and programs that are heavily skewed toward a negativity bias.

This pervasive negativity bias in our thought patterns has significant implications. As Earl Nightingale insightfully remarked, "Whatever we plant in our subconscious mind and nourish with repetition and emotion will one day become a reality." If the seeds we plant are predominantly negative, the outcomes are likely to be negative. As we have seen through the placebo effect what we think and believe can affect our bodies.

This negative thought dynamic could partially explain why, since 1988, the use of antidepressant medications has surged by 400%, and why mental health issues have escalated to unprecedented levels. The challenge, then, is to become more aware of these non-conscious processes and to actively influence them towards more positive, empowering patterns, potentially transforming our mental health and well-being.

The Amazing Nervous System

The human nervous system is a complex, highly organized control panel coordinating everything we do. It affects our ability to move around as well as sense what is happening in and around us. The nervous system is divided into two main parts: the central nervous system (CNS) and the peripheral nervous system (PNS).

Although the brain may not be the boss of everything, it is still pretty amazing and is the headquarters of our central nervous system consisting of the brain and the spinal cord. The brain processes all the information we receive from our senses and regulates our bodily functions, as well as helps us think, feel, and remember things. The spinal cord is a pathway that carries messages between the brain and the rest of the body and coordinates reflexes.

The peripheral nervous system includes all of the neural elements outside of the central nervous system and is divided into two parts: the somatic nervous system which is responsible for voluntary movements such as moving our arms and legs and the autonomic nervous system which controls involuntary bodily functions that we usually don't think about, like our heart beating and digestion. The autonomic nervous system is further subdivided into the sympathetic (which prepares the body for 'fight or flight' responses to react quickly in emergencies) and the parasympathetic (which supports 'rest and digest' and restorative activities) nervous systems.

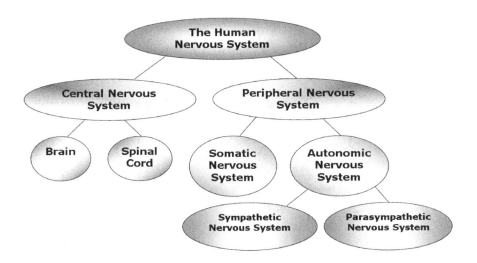

The nervous system's remarkable ability to detect, interpret, and respond to changes both inside and outside the body is essential for our survival. It plays a key role in adapting our behaviors to different situations and maintaining balance, or homeostasis, in our body. This means it helps keep our internal environment stable, even when external conditions change. For example, it can trigger sweating to cool us down or shivering to warm us up, depending on the temperature. This adaptability and responsiveness make the nervous system vital in managing our body's responses and ensuring we can thrive in a variety of environments.

The Autonomic Nervous System and the Breath-Brain Connection

The autonomic nervous system controls many of the body's automatic functions, like heart rate, blood pressure, metabolism, temperature regulation, salivation, and digestion. Consisting of its two principal branches, the sympathetic and parasympathetic

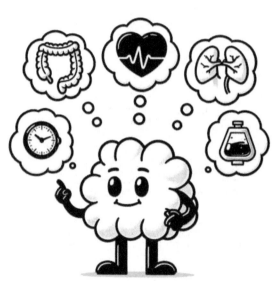

nervous systems, the autonomic nervous system makes sure our body functions smoothly while responding to what is happening around us and keeping us safe.

When learning about new medical terms, I always find it useful to understand where the words come from.

"Autonomic" is used in reference to the portion of the nervous system that is automatic – we are not able to consciously control it because it is involuntary.

"Sympathetic nervous system" was coined in the 17th century by an English physician, Thomas Willis, who believed its function was to coordinate the body's responses to stress and emotion in a sympathetic or caring manner (this always seemed strange to me because "fight or flight" doesn't seem "sympathetic", but an easy way to remember it is "sympathetic" starts with "S" and so does "stress" and "survival").

"Parasympathetic" simply adds a "para" in front of "sympathetic" meaning "beside" (my memory technique for remembering "parasympathetic" is it starts with a "P" and so does "peace"). So parasympathetic essentially means "alongside the sympathetic" to highlight its role as the counterpart to the sympathetic nervous system. Interestingly, the incredible importance of the parasympathetic nervous system has come to light in recent years and determines how well we are able to respond to stress.

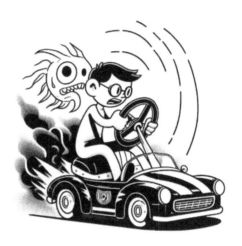

The sympathetic nervous system is like the gas pedal in a car – it revs up our body stress response and prepares us to deal with danger. When we are stressed or anxious, the sympathetic nervous system kicks into gear, causing our heart rate to increase, our muscles to tense up, and our breathing to become rapid and shallow. This is known as the "fight or flight" response, and it is designed to help us react quickly to threats. When the sympathetic nervous system activates, the body prioritizes survival over maintaining its usual balance and restorative functions because the main goal is to escape danger, rather than fixing any ongoing issues within the body. When a tiger is chasing you, escaping is more important than repairing damaged cells. An extended period of time in the sympathetic state because of chronic stress can lead to problems as the body never gets the chance to engage its restorative functions and doesn't get the opportunity to fix itself like it should. This can lead to the body breaking down over time.

On the flip side, the parasympathetic nervous system acts like a brake pedal, slowing us down and helping us relax once the danger is gone. When the parasympathetic nervous system is running the show, our heart rate slows, our muscles loosen up, and our breathing becomes slow and deep. This response, called the "rest and digest" mode, helps us bounce back from stress and bring our body back into balance by maintaining homeostasis, the body's natural equilibrium. It gives our body a chance to repair and recharge, getting us ready for whatever comes next. When our parasympathetic nervous system works well, it lets our body rest and repair itself so we can be ready for the next challenge. It also turns out that advanced mammalian parasympathetic input of the nervous system allows us to better interact with others in social engagement which we will discuss in more detail in a moment.

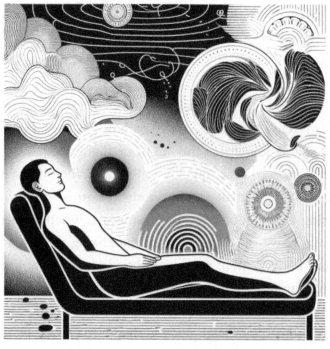

The Polyvagal Theory

Building on our basic understanding of the nervous system, let's investigate the Polyvagal Theory, a model developed by Dr. Stephen Porges which offers deeper insights into how our body responds to stress and forms social connections. This theory goes beyond the traditional view of the autonomic nervous system, which used to be seen as a simple balance between the "fight or flight" response of the sympathetic system and the "rest and digest" function of the parasympathetic system. The medical community originally believed it was like a light switch – when one was on, the other was off. However, the autonomic nervous system is far more layered than previously thought where there are three main parts that can be partially on or off in a gradient fashion at the same time.

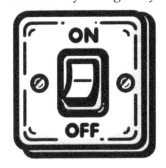

The Polyvagal Theory introduces a third component of the autonomic nervous system, which is managed by a specific part of the 10th cranial nerve called the vagus nerve which is a pivotal player in the autonomic nervous system. The vagus nerve oversees numerous vital functions like heart rate, digestion, and breathing.

In the Polyvagal Theory, the older, reptilian part of the vagus nerve, known as the Dorsal Vagal Complex (DVC), triggers a "freeze" or "faint" shutdown response when it perceives an overwhelming threat where neither fight nor flight is a viable option, acting as a protective mechanism during overwhelming threats. Conversely, the more evolved, mammalian part of the vagus nerve, the Ventral Vagal Complex (VVC), is associated with social communication, facial expressions, vocalization, and self-soothing behaviors. It promotes a sense of calm and fosters interactive connections, enabling social engagement and a sense of safety. It helps control heart rate and breathing in response to social situations felt to be nonthreatening. The Polyvagal Theory sheds light on how our responses to stress are structured.

As I have now introduced several new medical terms, here are some memory techniques and word origin information to help make learning easier. The term "poly" means "many," highlighting the varied influences of the vagus nerve, which is an incredibly long nerve and extends throughout the body. The vagus nerve's name derives from the Latin for "wandering," indicating its extensive reach. A memory mnemonic to remember the vagus nerve is **VAGUS** = Vital Avenue Generating Upbeat and Shutdown. "Vital Avenue" refers to this very long and crucial pathway throughout the body. "Generating Upbeat and Shutdown" refers to the VVC which is upbeat and happy as we interact with others and to the DVC which results in shutdown.

The "D" of the Dorsal Vagus Complex (DVC) stands for "dorsal" which comes from the Latin word "dorsum," meaning "back." It refers to the part of the vagus nerve originating closer to the back side of the brainstem. A memory technique to remember what "dorsal" means is to imagine carrying a door on your back. Some of you 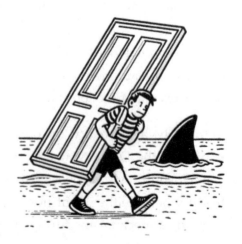 may also know that the "dorsal fin" on a shark's back is what sticks out of the water and can terrify you into a state of shock. Also, sharks have the DVC but do not have the VVC because they are not mammals.

The "V" of the Ventral Vagus Complex stands for "ventral" which comes from the Latin word "venter," meaning "belly" or "stomach." It refers to the part of the vagus nerve which is nearer the front side of the brainstem. A memory technique for remembering "Ventral" is "Valuing friendship upfront" which helps you remember the front side of the body as well as its role in social interaction.

The Ventral Vagal Complex (VVC) is a relatively recent evolutionary addition found only in mammals, and is crucial for social engagement and self-soothing. When activated, it allows us to connect with others, fostering empathy, joy, and secure relationships. It helps to regulate stress and fosters calm connection states, enabling productive interaction with others and feelings of safety. It is our "happy place."

Ventral Vagal Complex (VVC)
Newer Part of the Autonomic Nervous System
Social Engagement and Self-Soothing
The Happy Place

Sympathetic Nervous System
Fight or Flight
Responds to Danger

Dorsal Vagal Complex (DVC)
Older Part of the Autonomic Nervous System
Freeze or Faint
Kicks in when Fight or Flight are not Options
Can become chronically engaged with constant stress or unresolved trauma

---

In the presence of danger, we transition from the VVC to a state of sympathetic activation—geared for immediate physical action. This includes rapid heartbeat, dilated pupils, and heightened alertness. Our muscles tighten and get ready to move while our body revs up energy to face the impending threat. But what if fighting or running away is not an option?

If escape or confrontation is not an option, the DVC takes over, leading to a shutdown or "playing possum," hoping the threat passes. This part of the nervous system is felt to be around 500 million years old, so it is about 100 million years older than the sympathetic nervous system and 300 million years older than the VVC. The DVC results in immobilization by either fainting or faking death by freezing.

When we are in the sympathetic state, it is highly energy-consuming and unsustainable for long durations. Prolonged exposure leads to excessive cortisol which is harmful to the heart. If we are trapped in this sympathetic activated state for too long, the body gears down to the DVC to manage stress through immobilization. This is why people in a state of shock often seemed eerily calm because of the

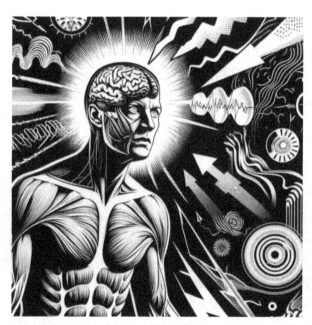

DVC shutdown reaction.

Chronic activation of these stress responses—either through ongoing sympathetic arousal (typical in chronic stress) or DVC activation (common after trauma that has not been processed)—keeps our bodies in a constant state of survival. This can lead to heightened pain sensitivity, altered perceptions of the world as threatening, and impaired social connections. When we are in survival state, with chronically tight muscles, increased heart rate, and increased blood pressure, we have decreased energy and poor digestion because our focus is on safety and not on homeostasis and restorative functions to keep ourselves going. It affects us emotionally and physically. This is not about changing your thoughts. This is physiology. These systems are hundreds of millions of years old and they do not know that language exists, so thinking a positive thought is not going to change them. We cannot have a rational conversation with them. The way to access them is through the physical body, physical sensation, and disrupting these neuronal processes to bring us back to a state of balance and connection, governed by the VVC. This is why Breathwork is a shortcut to healing our chronic stress and resolving our unprocessed traumas.

Brain–Heart Coherence

Now that we have examined the inner workings of the brain and the nervous system, let's look at how the brain and heart interact when they are synched up in coherence. This connection, known as brain-heart coherence, involves the state of synchronization when the heart's rhythmic patterns and the brain's electrical activity are harmonized. It happens when the heart's signals of a safe and happy environment influence the brain's electrical signals to align. As we delve deeper, we will explore the definition of coherence and how our emotional state and feelings can significantly affect the synchronicity connection, influencing both clear thinking and emotional resilience.

The definition of a coherent system is a complex system with many parts working together in harmony with energy efficiency where the sum of the parts leads to a greater whole. A coherent system is like a well organized team where all the players work together smoothly, making everything run efficiently. Think of it as a big puzzle where every piece fits just right, creating something incredible when they all come together. Coherence can be in an individual organism on a personal level, but it can also be on a bigger social or even global level. When everything is working in harmony and is aligned in high energy efficiency - that is coherence.

Contrary to past misconceptions within the medical community as we discussed earlier, the brain does not reign supreme over the body. There is a complicated neuronal and hormonal system in which all the parts of the body work together and communicate back and forth with each other. The heart emerges as one of the most prominent communicators, conveying a wealth of information to the brain, and actually sends more messages to the brain than it receives. The heart has its own logic and acts independently from the brain. Not only does the heart not obey the brain, but it has perception and can tell the brain what to do – especially in the case of processing emotions.

Brain–heart coherence refers to the state where the activity and rhythms of the brain and the heart are harmoniously synchronized. The brain and the heart are connected through various pathways, including the autonomic nervous system, which regulates involuntary physiological processes. Perhaps some of the most exciting research findings in the field of brain-heart coherence are its relationship between heart rate variability (HRV) and emotional well-being.

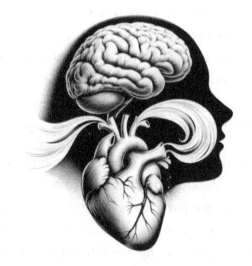

Heart Rate Variability or HRV

Central to understanding this communication between the heart and brain is heart rate variability (HRV) which is a key indicator of the autonomic nervous system's responsiveness and stability. It reflects how well the body can maintain homeostasis or internal balance in response to what is going on outside as well as inside our bodies. High HRV is generally considered a marker of good health and resilience, indicating a strong ability to adapt to stress. The more variable our HRV, the more capable we are to handle the next challenge.

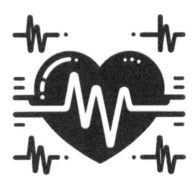

Most people know what heart rate is – it is the number of times our heart beats in a minute. Heart rate variability goes a step further and measures the change from one heartbeat to the next. This beat to beat variation is called heart rate variability or HRV. If the HRV were the same between each heartbeat, then it would be like a metronome used in music where the beat happens always at the same time interval. There will be no heart rhythm but simply a steady heart rate. Thirty to fifty years ago, physicians were taught that a sign of good health was a steady heart rate which is totally wrong. In fact, if we lose this natural heart rate variability it is a strong predictor of future health problems including early mortality.

This ability to vary the time between heartbeats enables us to effectively accommodate to stressful situations in our environment, and it is an excellent marker of our abilities to adapt. Heart rate variability is our best marker of aging. We have greater heart rate variability when we are younger, and it decreases as we age. The decline in HRV observed with advancing age signifies not only the natural progression of time but also underscores potential health risk. Diminished HRV emerges as an indicator of imbalance in our system. It is implicated in a spectrum of ailments ranging from metabolic disorders to cardiovascular diseases. Low heart rate variability is strongly associated with more disease such as diabetes, chronic lung disease, heart and blood pressure problems, but the number one cause of low heart rate variability is chronic stress.

Chronic stress emerges as a potent disruptor of HRV, underscoring the detrimental impact of prolonged stress on physiological resilience. We are decreasing our nervous system's ability to adapt to change because of the long term exhaustion from always being stressed. When we are always stressed, our nervous system gets worn out and cannot adapt well to changes. This means our body struggles more to bounce back and stay healthy. One way we can become aware and eventually improve our HRV is by monitoring it. There are many free apps for smart phones that measure HRV. Check them out.

Heart rate variability is more than just a simple measure; it shows how the brain, heart, and the body's automatic nerve system work together. This gives us a full picture of how well our body's systems are connected and working. HRV isn't just about the heart; it also involves the brain and the connections between the heart and brain. It is an integrated system. They all have to be working properly to generate a healthy heart rate variability. As a dynamic metric reflecting the interdependence of multiple factors, HRV embodies the essence of coherence, providing a window into the intricate dance of life's rhythms. Heart rate variability is an excellent measure to show the complete integrated system of our bodies. It is a helpful tool because it shows the teamwork between different parts of our body, offering a glimpse into the complex ways we handle life's ups and downs as it shows how our entire body system works together.

The Heart and Emotions

HRV is a particularly significant measure when considering the heart-brain connection in relation to emotions. In the early 1990s, researchers made a fascinating discovery: our heart's activity can tell us a lot about how we are feeling. It turned out to be a more reliable indicator of our emotional state than even brain scans. A higher 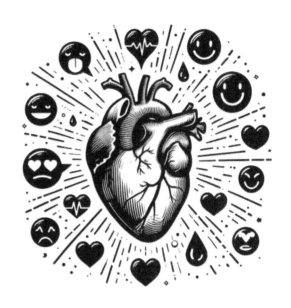 HRV indicates a more adaptable heart, capable of efficient responses to stress and emotional stimuli. Positive emotions are associated with a pattern of smooth, wavelike heart rhythms that enhance coherence between the heart and brain, improving energy, clarity, and problem-solving abilities. Conversely, negative emotions can lead to erratic, disordered heart rhythms, which can disrupt brain function, impair cognitive processes, and lead to feelings of discomfort or anxiety.

Studies focused on positive feelings like "appreciation" and "gratitude" showed that when we feel these emotions deeply, our hearts produce a different identifiable rhythm. This unique pattern of heart activity is now known as coherence. Since the 1990s, over

400 studies have explored this connection, revealing that when we are in a positive emotional state, our body systems work together in a more synchronized and efficient way, creating coherence. We are able to measure blood pressure, breathing rhythms, heart rate rhythms, intestinal rhythms, and brain waves and have discovered they have become more connected and ordered working together. When we are happy, our body works more optimally like a well-oiled machine.

Emotions can significantly affect the patterns of heart rate variability, and conversely, the heart can send signals to the brain that influence emotional processing. Positive emotions tend to increase HRV, leading to greater synchronization between the heart and brain, enhancing cognitive function like attention, perception, and problem solving. Increased coherence between the heart and the brain is associated with better emotional regulation, lower stress levels, enhanced mental clarity and decision-making capacity and overall better health outcomes.

Happy Emotions Lead to Coherence

The HeartMath Institute has contributed to this research and developed techniques to help people achieve coherence, even in the midst of everyday stressors. Various practices, such as mindfulness, meditation, and focused breathing exercises, are believed to enhance brain-heart coherence. These practices can help shift the body's balance from sympathetic to parasympathetic VVC dominance, promoting a state of calm, reducing stress, and improving physiological efficiency. Using practical methods to shift into coherence right in the moment even when life throws us curveballs, like traffic jams or difficult interactions, we can regulate our emotions and maintain our composure, ultimately enhancing our brain function and overall well-being.

Let's take an example of a man who is a longtime meditator who would meditate every morning and find his place of Zen, but then would experience road rage as someone cuts him off in traffic on his way to work. Despite the peaceful beginning to his day, he would arrive at work frustrated and irritable. These feelings of frustration begin a biochemical cascade in his body of stress hormones that deplete his energy and create incoherent rhythms in his heart and brain that will affect him for hours in the future. If the frustration and chronic stress become a daily pattern, this can affect him for the rest of his life.

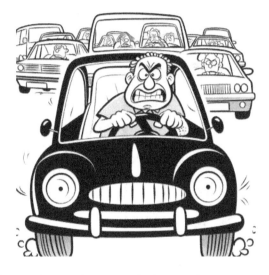

Most of us do not know how to shift to coherence by an act of our will. We fall victim to our emotions and circumstances. The key is noticing we are hooked and being able to shift into coherence in the moment we are in the traffic jams, getting phone calls, dealing with difficult people, and facing all of those challenges that confront us in daily life. To facilitate better brain function, we need a wider repertoire of choices to self-regulate and maintain our emotional composure. We need to know how to shift our emotional state at will – we need the remote control to inner calm. Luckily, our breath is the key.

The Different Rhythms of Coherence

In simpler terms, your body has various rhythms, like brain waves, heartbeats, blood pressure, breathing rate, and intestinal movements. These rhythms fluctuate but can sync up perfectly, like notes in a musical chord striking together. When this synchronization happens, your heart rate variability (HRV) improves, which is great for your longevity. This state of coherence, where everything works together harmoniously, is often triggered by positive emotions and is incredibly beneficial for your health.

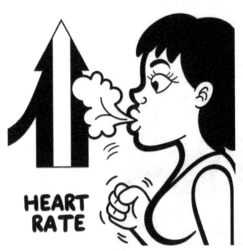

HEART RATE

When you inhale, your heart speeds up. When you exhale, it slows down. This means your breathing pattern directly influences your heart rate variability. The deeper and more regularly you breathe, the greater these changes in heart rate variability become. By examining HRV, we can actually measure how deep and how often someone is breathing. The rate and depth of our breath directly communicates with the heart to reveal our emotional state.

Breathing plays a crucial role in getting us into this cozy coherence zone. We cannot control all the circumstances in our lives, but we can control our breath. We can consciously intervene with it. We can choose to breathe slower and deeper into the diaphragm which helps to calm our nervous system and reduce the release of stress hormones like adrenaline or cortisol. Our breath remote control allows us to change our emotional state at will.

Brain Synchronization

Information travels from the heart to the brainstem and then reaches the thalamus, a critical part of the brain responsible for many jobs, including synchronizing the brain's electrical activity. For the brain to work well and function consciously, its electrical signals need to be in sync. This doesn't mean that all parts of the brain are doing the same thing at once; rather, it means that the brain's activities are well-coordinated. When the brain's electrical activity is synchronized, it means that the various neuronal circuits are firing in a coordinated pattern that optimizes brain function and promotes mental health and well-being. When the brain's electrical activity is in sync, the different brain circuits fire together in a pattern that makes the brain work best. This state of harmony in brain activity is critical for effective functioning and responsiveness to the environment. The brain can function well and react properly to what's happening around us.

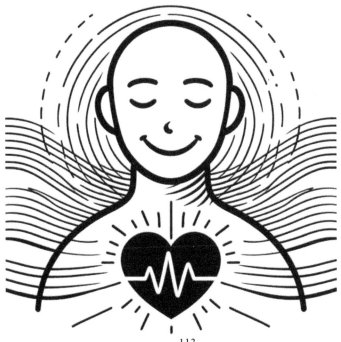

When we feel frustrated or impatient, we naturally experience incoherent rhythms. Our breathing changes to a shallower, erratic rhythm which tells the heart that "All is not right with the world." The heart then communicates this disharmony to the thalamus which disrupts its ability to ensure the brain's overall connectivity is coordinated. The brain is not synchronized. As a result, when we're angry or anxious, this incoherence leads to disorganized brain activity. In this agitated state, we are less able to focus, solve problems, perform complicated tasks, or react quickly in threatening situations. We are not on our A game.

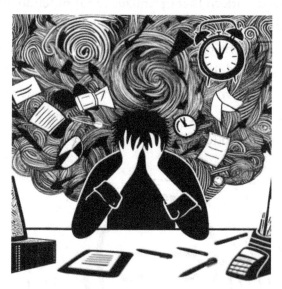

Conversely, when a coherent rhythm reaches the thalamus which was created from more positive emotions in response to our breath and HRV, it boosts the brain's ability to synchronize its activity. A coherent heart rhythm improves reaction times and emotional regulation, enhancing the brain's capacity to plan and think ahead. Often times when we practice coherent breathing, the answers to previously difficult questions will pop into our heads. In coherence, our brain is synchronized and solving problems becomes easier. Coherence enhances the brain's performance.

The Amygdala: Familiar or Not

Another important part of the brain that affects how we feel stress is the amygdala. It's a small, almond-shaped part of the brain that helps manage our emotions, react to fear, remember things, make decisions, and understand social situations. Recent studies have shown us more about the amygdala, especially how it helps us tell the difference between things we know and things we don't know. It determines what is familiar and what is not. This function is crucial because it helps us navigate our environment more safely and efficiently by quickly assessing whether something is known and safe or unknown and potentially a threat.

The amygdala processes sensory inputs from the environment and compares them to stored memories. If something matches as familiar, previously encountered, and safe, then the amygdala can trigger a recognition response leading to a more relaxed and less stressed state as the brain perceives less threat. When the amygdala encounters something new or unfamiliar, it can activate a heightened state of alertness. This involves preparing the body to respond to potential threats through the activation of stress responses, like the "fight or flight" mechanism. This heightened alertness is crucial for survival of potential danger.

To figure out what is familiar and what is not, the amygdala needs to compare new experiences with what it already knows. Different emotions like frustration, anxiety, compassion, and sadness each have unique patterns that the amygdala recognizes. The amygdala compares the current heart rhythm to past emotional patterns—like those associated with feeling good or feeling stressed—to decide what we are experiencing now and whether we are safe or not. For example, it can recognize emotions of appreciation, stress, or happiness. When the heart rhythm is calm and steady, the amygdala might conclude that we are safe and that the body feels good.

Often, people who have chronic stress, long-term anxiety, or a history of significant trauma may find that their amygdala marks many things as unsafe, even if they aren't. This usually relates to deep-seated, unconscious patterns formed in childhood. This is why some people might feel uncomfortable just one minute into practicing coherence breathing. They might say they don't like it or that it doesn't feel right. Understanding how the amygdala works helps us see why this happens. If the amygdala isn't used to a calm pattern because of long-term stress, it doesn't recognize "calm" as safe. This causes a mismatch, making the brain feel uneasy. It takes time to get used to this calm state and feel comfortable with it. I personally experienced something similar to this when I first started practicing coherent breathing which we will get into shortly.

The Resonant Frequency: Coherence Breathing

The resonant frequency in coherence breathing refers to the optimal breathing rate at which an individual's heart rate variability (HRV) maximizes, leading to increased synchronization between the cardiovascular, respiratory, and nervous systems. It is all about the ratio where the inhale time equals the exhale time to create balance. Although you can use any equal number of seconds for the inhale and exhale, research finds that one inhale every 5.5 seconds and one exhale every 5.5 seconds is consistent with the most coherent rhythmic breathing. This is six breaths per minute. Because there is a slight pause at the top and a slight pause at the bottom, we can simplify the 5.5 seconds by breathing five seconds in and five seconds out. The brain and heart naturally like to oscillate at this rhythm because it causes a coherent state.

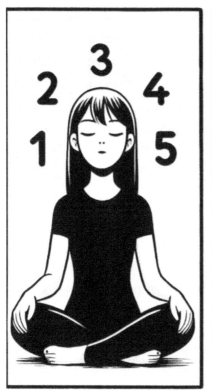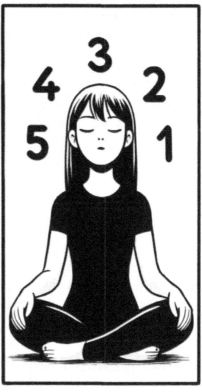

Try it out. Try breathing in to a count of five. One, two, three, four, five. Then out for a count of five. On the exhale, I like to count backwards which seems to relax me even more. Five, four, three, two, one. Keep breathing in this pattern for at least five minutes to really see a difference. Depending on CO2 tolerance, a five second inhale and exhale may be too difficult to start as it was for me. That's okay. Count to five on the inhale; count down from five on the exhale with the same pattern – it is okay if to count a little faster than a second as long as the rate is the same for the inhale and exhale. As CO2 tolerance increases, a full five second inhale and exhale will be possible. For fun, try measuring your HRV before and after doing this exercise.

As I mentioned, coherent breathing felt uncomfortable to me to start. My baseline Breath Hold Time (BHT) was only 12 seconds so my CO_2 tolerance was pretty low at baseline. I focused on having the same time on the inhale as on the exhale and not worrying about whether each count was a second or not. Inhaling is sympathetic input (heart rate goes up) and exhaling is parasympathetic (heart rate slows down). I found that I was fine breathing in – 1, 2, 3, 4, 5 – but on the exhale, I started feeling like I needed to breathe on the 2 of the - 5, 4, 3, 2, 1. Allowing my exhale to be as long as my inhale felt so strange as my pattern for years was chronic stress in the sympathetic state with longer inhales than exhales. Understanding the science behind this and witnessing my body's chronic sympathetic state, helped me stick with it and after only a few rounds, it became comfortable and quite calming. I often breathe in this pattern in the car or any time I am bored and think about it. Seeing how we can incorporate coherent breathing into our everyday lives will make a tremendous difference in combating chronic stress. Balance out those ratios.

Achieving Coherence

Always the first step is to become aware. Being aware and attentive to our feelings and bodily sensations is crucial. What is going on in the body and nervous system? Be curious about the quality of the emotion. Is this emotion depleting or does it replenish? Is it draining or rejuvenating? As soon as we become aware that we are in a negative, incoherent emotional state, then we are able to do something about it. We cannot fix something of which we are not aware.

Breathing is the next step. For centuries, breathing techniques have been a staple advice for calming down. We often hear, "take a deep breath," when tensions run high. Oftentimes we cannot even discuss what is bothering us until we have managed to calm down first. Calming ourselves helps us listen and communicate better about our troubles.

If someone cuts us off in traffic, deep slow belly breathing can reduce the intensity of our reaction. It helps soothe our nervous system, slowing our heart rate and decreasing the release of stress hormones like adrenaline or epinephrine. The release of stress hormones is not completely prevented, however, as the cascade leading to incoherence in our system has initiated. Slow deep belly breathing doesn't entirely eliminate the negative feelings like anxiety or frustration, but it does reduce their intensity, setting the stage for us to change our emotional state. Calming down is great, however, the goal isn't just to calm down; it is to shift from that unpleasant, stressful emotional state of incoherence to a more positive state that fosters coherence. This involves the next step of focusing on your heart space while coherent breathing (5 seconds in and

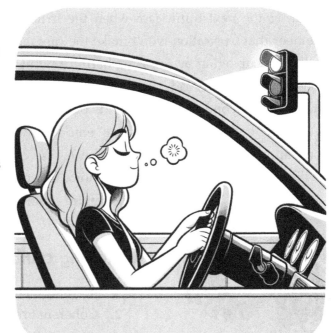

5 seconds out). Draw attention away from the racing thoughts in the head and feel the heart. Feel the breath expanding in the heart.

Where we focus our attention causes changes in our body. This is what the biofeedback industry is founded on.

After we begin coherent breathing, we turn our focus on our heart space and then begin the final step of achieving coherence—generating a feeling of gratitude or appreciation. These emotions are some of the easiest positive emotions for us to create at will. We imagine a time in our life when we felt most grateful. See it; feel it; hear it; smell it. Step into that memory of appreciation and gratitude. It is easiest to do these steps with our eyes closed, but when doing so would not be safe, eyes open will still work. I have successfully done these steps while driving and even in front of triggering people without their even knowing. Doing this process for just 5 minutes can help us achieve a harmonious state.

So, during the next traffic jam when the irritation begins to boil, remember that frustration won't make the cars move any faster, but it will speed up aging by releasing harmful hormones leading to an incoherent state. Instead, we can adopt a coherent breathing pattern—five seconds in, five seconds out—and steer our attention toward the heart while generating emotions like gratitude and appreciation to bring us back to coherence. We cannot make all the cars disappear, but we can make the choice to respond in a way that

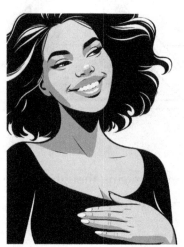

is better for both our physical and mental health.

Achieving Coherence

1. Become aware
2. Coherent breathing (5 seconds in, 5 seconds out)
3. Bring focus to your heart
4. Generate emotion of gratitude or appreciation

Feeling Good is Good for Us

It's widely understood that stress is harmful to our health, both from a scientific standpoint and as common knowledge. However, what we often overlook is how feeling good is good for us. Feeling good is beneficial to our health. Many of us even feel guilty for enjoying ourselves or experiencing positive emotions. Society has brainwashed us into believing that feeling good is selfish. Inflicting guilt and self-abuse when we take the time for self-care and self-soothing is completely counterproductive. Negative emotions deplete us. Feeling love, compassion, appreciation, and kindness not only feels good—these emotions are actually beneficial for our health and can significantly impact our longevity. We cannot be here for others emotionally or physically, if we cut our lives short with chronic stress. Sticking around by feeling positive emotions helps not only ourselves but everyone else as well.

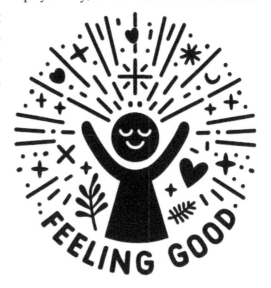

Interestingly, the heart responds differently to each emotion, producing unique frequencies for each emotional state. By examining patterns in heart rate variability (HRV), it's possible to identify not only the specific emotion someone is experiencing, but also the intensity of that emotion. Positive emotions replenish us, unlike negative emotions, which drain our energy and can accelerate aging because of the stress they generate. Understanding and fostering positive emotions is crucial, not just for individual well-being but also for societal and global health.

Our Magnetic Field

An electrocardiogram, commonly known as an EKG or ECG, measures the electrical activity of the heart. The heart is the strongest source of electrical energy in the body, and where there is electrical energy; there is also a magnetic field which we can measure with a device called a magnetometer. This magnetic field extends at least a meter around the body—it may go further but our instruments can only detect so far. This magnetic field generated by the heart's electrical activity can be measured and even used to determine a person's emotional state, as it carries distinct patterns

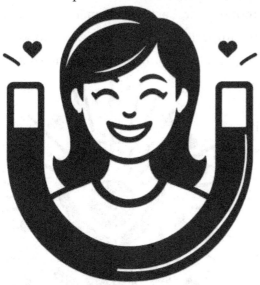

influenced by emotions. The magnetic field is a carrier of information modified by emotions and probably many other factors still being investigated. We know that we emit a magnetic field into the space around us, and this field carries information related to our emotions and heart rhythms. But does this field have a measurable impact on others? Research says yes. Our nervous systems are finely tuned to detect these biological magnetic fields generated by others. We can literally feel the emotional and physiological states of those around us, influenced by both their hearts and brains.

Studies have shown that our nervous systems not only detect these fields but are affected by them. When someone is in a coherent state, emitting a more orderly magnetic field, it can positively influence those around them, often without their conscious awareness. This phenomenon is reflected in our everyday language—phrases like "the tension was so thick, you could cut it with a knife" or "it feels good to be around so-and-so" hint at our ability to sense and be affected by the fields of others.

This goes beyond verbal and non-verbal communication like tone of voice or body language. There is a vital, energetic interaction happening all the time between individuals and within groups. This inter-energetic communication is not only fascinating but potentially more impactful than we previously understood, influencing and uplifting others based on the quality of our personal energy field.

Incoherence Causes Problems

Research indicates that 70% to 80% of mistakes in business and healthcare result from communication errors. These issues often stem from what's known as energetic miscommunication—a mismatch between what's being said and the emotional energy being transmitted. This phenomenon can be observed in everyday interactions, particularly during heated conversations.

Consider a scenario involving two colleagues, Sarah and Jim, who are discussing a critical project. Sarah is speaking calmly and using neutral words, but inside, she is frustrated and anxious about an unrelated personal issue. Her magnetic field, which conveys her true emotional state, radiates these feelings. Jim, on the other hand, senses Sarah's frustration not through her words but through the energy she is emitting. He starts to feel defensive and anxious, believing that Sarah is unhappy with his contributions to the project. Although Sarah's words are neutral, the emotional charge in her magnetic field causes Jim to react as if she had directly criticized him.

This discrepancy between spoken words and the emotional signals we emit is a significant source of miscommunication. Even if we try to appear cheerful with a forced smile while feeling distressed, our true emotions often come across more strongly to others through our energy field. The magnetic field can be more powerful than the words we are speaking.

To illustrate, let's look at another example involving a healthcare setting. Dr. Miller, a seasoned physician, is discussing a treatment

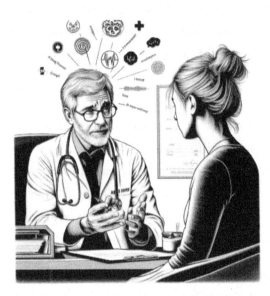

plan with a patient, Emily. Dr. Miller is stressed because of a backlog of patients and administrative issues, but he tries to maintain a calm demeanor. Despite his efforts, his underlying stress permeates his communication. Emily picks up on this stress and becomes anxious, doubting the doctor's

confidence in the treatment plan. This leads to a lack of trust and potentially poorer adherence to the prescribed regimen, even though Dr. Miller's verbal instructions were clear and accurate.

By achieving coherence within ourselves through emotional awareness, breathing techniques, and managing our emotions, we can positively influence those around us. When we are coherent, we are more present in the moment we are actually in, and our emotional state is aligned with our thoughts and words, creating a more harmonious energy field. This coherence can be contagious, potentially helping others to align their own energies.

For example, consider a manager, Lisa, who has mastered emotional coherence. She regularly practices mindfulness and Breathwork, ensuring her emotional state is balanced. During a stressful team meeting, Lisa remains calm and composed, her energy radiating a sense of stability and confidence. Her team members, who might be feeling stressed or anxious, begin to pick up on Lisa's coherent energy. As a result, the overall atmosphere of the meeting shifts towards a more productive and less tense environment. The team is better able to focus on problem-solving and collaboration, rather than being bogged down by misaligned emotions and miscommunication.

However, it is essential to recognize that while we can offer coherence, we can't force someone to accept it. People must be open to change; if they choose to remain in a state of anger or upset, they will. For instance, if one of Lisa's team members, Jake, is determined to stay upset about a recent policy change, Lisa's coherence may not immediately influence him. Jake needs to be 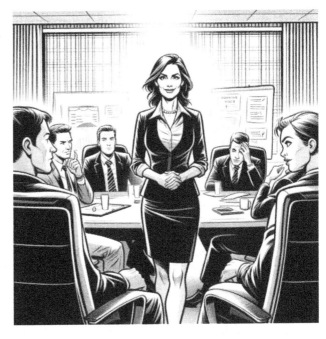 receptive to the positive energy for it to have an effect. But if he is open, Lisa's coherent presence can uplift him, helping him to see the situation more clearly and respond more effectively.

By achieving coherence within ourselves through emotional awareness, breathing techniques, and managing our emotions, we can positively influence those around us. When we are coherent, we can project this state, potentially helping others to align their own energies. It reduces the risk of miscommunication caused by energetic discrepancies and can create a more positive and productive environment in both personal and professional settings. By being aware of our emotional states and using techniques to manage them, we not only improve our own well-being but also positively influence those around us.

Global Coherence

Imagine a world where everyone achieves coherence; this concept is known as global coherence. The HeartMath Institute is actively working towards this by setting up magnetic monitoring stations worldwide to track the Earth's magnetic fields. Interestingly, one of the Earth's natural frequencies is 0.1 Hz, which matches the frequency of a coherent human heart. This suggests a deep connection between personal coherence and global harmony.

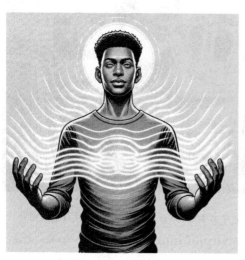

Global coherence begins with individual efforts. By focusing on regulating our emotions and maintaining personal coherence, we contribute to changing the world. Each of us controls our own energy field, influencing everyone we encounter. We can actively think about what we are contributing to the collective energy field: What am I radiating from my personal field right now?

What am I feeding the field? Am I promoting kindness, compassion, and appreciation? Or am I adding frustration, anxiety, and stress because I am overwhelmed by daily tasks? Changing our personal field is a choice we can make moment to moment.

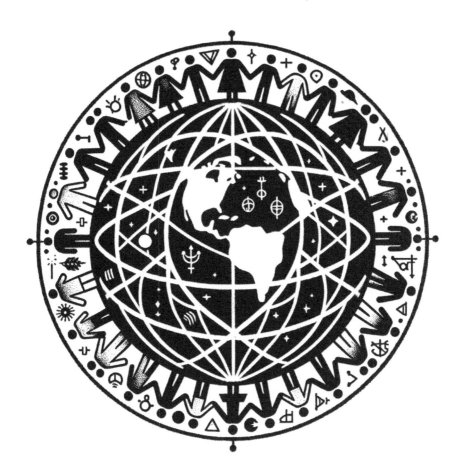

The significance of our contributions cannot be overstated. The more of us who learn to cultivate a coherent field by choosing to infuse our environments with love, compassion, kindness, and gratitude, the more we enhance not only our own health and longevity but also facilitate a shift in global consciousness.

6
BREATH: THE SILENT HEALER WITHIN

"Breath is the key to unlocking the full potential of our body, mind, and spirit. Through conscious breathing, we can access deep states of relaxation and healing."

- Dr. Andrew Weil

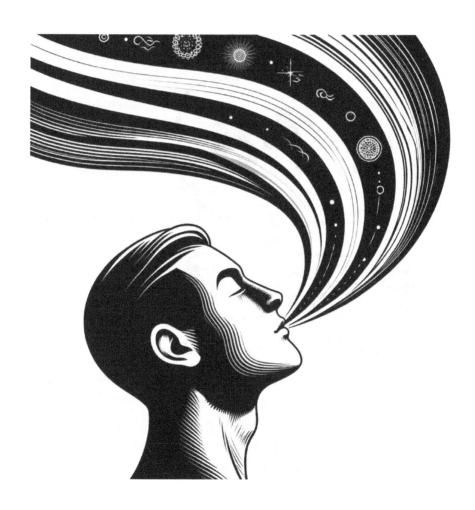

A Transformational Journey: Unlocking Healing Through Somatic Breathwork

Before we explore traditional Breathwork practices geared towards fostering long-term change for managing chronic stress in the next chapter, let's first examine the transformative power of Somatic Release and Transformational Breathwork. These techniques offer the potential for instantaneous change and profoundly altered my life in a single 90-minute session.

My journey into Breathwork began unexpectedly. With a background as a board-certified Addiction Medicine specialist, I

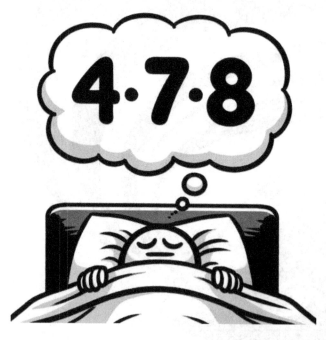

sought to learn new methods to aid my patients struggling with anxiety. This led me to a training conference to become a facilitator in Somatic Release Breathwork. I enrolled without prior experience or knowledge about what I was about to encounter. Initially, I imagined learning straightforward techniques like the 4-7-8 breathing method popularized by Dr. Andrew Weil for managing insomnia. However, the reality was starkly different and infinitely more immediately impactful.

The conference included multiple full days of instruction, culminating in my first Somatic Release Breathwork session. Conducted in a large conference room with a hundred other participants, this was not the way most people first experience Breathwork. That 90-minute session was transformative, equating to 5 years of talk therapy. During that first session, I found myself expressing a spectrum of trapped emotions—screaming, crying, and uncontrollably laughing—without the need to verbalize or consciously recall past traumas. This spontaneous emotional release allowed me to confront and let go of deep-seated pains in a way I never thought possible.

This experience was a revelation. I felt like a new person. Despite years of conventional talk therapy, where I gained a cognitive understanding of my issues, the emotional residue remained unaddressed. Somatic Release Breathwork offered a direct pathway to healing, bypassing the need for cognitive processing. It seemed like a magic bullet, especially considering many of my addiction patients use substances not for euphoria but for numbness. Addressing  these underlying emotional traumas could potentially transform the approach to addiction treatment by focusing on the root causes rather than merely alleviating symptoms.

Inspired by the profound impact of my experience, I committed to advocating and integrating Breathwork into therapeutic practices globally. This method isn't just about learning to breathe; it's about learning to feel, heal, and ultimately, transform. For information on Breathwork journeys available to you, check out resources at the back of this book and on TheBreathMD.com.

Understanding Somatic Release Breathwork

The term "somatic" refers to the body. As we discussed in Chapter 2, a major contributor to chronic stress is the presence of unprocessed emotions and trapped traumas. Somatic Release Breathwork is designed to liberate these trapped energies from the body. Steven Jaggers, a master of a specific Somatic Release method known as The Soma+IQ Method, describes it as "an embodiment experience that moves you beyond your thinking mind, allowing for the release of unneeded, unprocessed energy in a safe environment." This process is aimed at enhancing life quality.

Research involving over 1,000 participants of this method has shown remarkable benefits: 91% reported increased resilience to stress, 77% experienced transformative dynamics in personal relationships, 89% observed improved emotional regulation, 93% noticed enhanced self-awareness and introspection, and 87% felt a significant boost in energy and vitality.

Somatic Release Breathwork employs a technique known as circular connected breathing, where there is no pause between inhalation and exhalation, helping to revitalize the connection between the mind and the body's inherent wisdom. Typically, each session lasts about an hour. The initial half involves deep, rhythmic breathing in and out through the mouth accompanied by activating music, while the latter half transitions to a more serene experience with nasal inhalation and mouth exhalation set to calming tunes. Throughout the session, there are several breath holds that often bring profound insights. The facilitator minimizes speaking, using only encouraging words and thought-provoking questions to guide the experience. In-person sessions may include gentle hand placements by the facilitator, but primarily, it's an intimate journey between you and your breath. The transformative power of these sessions often stems directly from this deep, personal engagement with the breathing process.

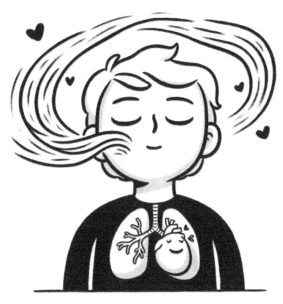

Jason's Story: The Consequences of Suppressed Anger

Jason had always struggled with his temper. One evening, a heated argument with his dad pushed him to the brink. He felt cornered, criticized, and like nothing he did was ever good enough. The interaction ended with him being yelled at, and he left the room feeling a deep sense of frustration and resentment. Unable to express his anger to his dad, Jason felt a storm brewing inside him. Back in his room, he saw the model plane he had been meticulously building for weeks. In a fit of rage, he smashed it to pieces. The brief release of anger left him feeling empty and even more upset. He reached for a joint, hoping it would numb the turmoil within him.

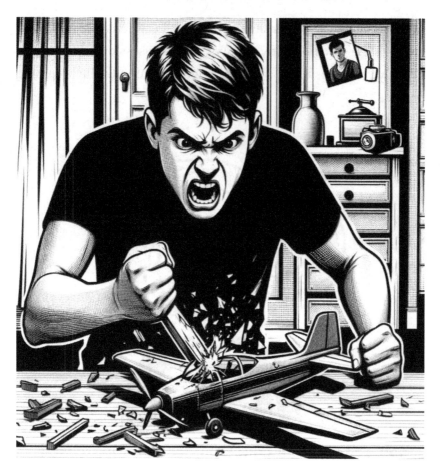

Later that night, he met up with a friend, but the unresolved anger from earlier in the day lingered. His friend, noticing his unusually sharp and snarky demeanor, tried to help, but Jason snapped at her. The evening ended in another argument, leaving Jason feeling guilty and regretful for hurting someone he cared about.

Jason's inability to express his anger directly and responsibly had led to a cascade of negative consequences. His unresolved emotions spilled over into other areas of his life, damaging his relationships and leaving him feeling more isolated and distressed.

The Alternative: Somatic Release Breathwork

If Jason had turned to Somatic Release Breathwork instead, the outcome might have been very different. Breathwork offers a safe space to process and release intense emotions like anger. In a Breathwork journey, Jason could have channeled his frustration through deep, intentional breathing exercises, allowing his body to fully experience and then release the pent-up anger. It is better to let the anger out on the mat than out into the world.

By engaging in Breathwork, Jason could have felt the physical sensations of his anger and let them go. This practice not only helps in releasing the immediate tension but also fosters a sense of inner peace and emotional regulation.

Incorporating Somatic Release Breathwork into his practice, Jason could transform his relationship with anger, learning to express it healthily and preventing the negative ripple effects on his life and relationships. Instead of smashing his model plane and hurting his friend, Jason could find peace on the mat, emerging calmer, more emotionally regulated and centered.

Exploring Transformational Breathwork: A Gateway to Deep Healing

Transformational Breathwork is a broad term that encompasses a variety of practices, often referred to collectively as Regenerative or Somatic Release Breathwork with guided mediations. Central to these practices is the concept of "conscious connected breathing," where there are no pauses between inhalations and exhalations, creating a continuous, looping breath pattern as described earlier. This method is highly regarded for its lasting effect on psychological and emotional healing, as it facilitates access to the subconscious mind, releases trapped emotions and traumas, and aids in rewiring the brain.

Transformational Breathwork is named for its profound impact, making it a standout among healing methods. It provides immediate relief for some, serving as a quick switch to an improved feeling state. There simply are not many treatments out there with the ability to affect such rapid change for the better.

While similar to Somatic Release Breathwork in its use of conscious connected breath, Transformational Breathwork incorporates additional elements such as guided imagery and affirmations to reframe limiting beliefs that are connected with the release of traumas. The 9D version of this practice, developed by Brian Kelly—a renowned Breathworker based in Bali—integrates diverse auditory stimuli, including binaural beats and subliminal messages, to enrich the healing experience. This version can be practiced privately, making it accessible for personal transformation within one's own bedroom.

According to Brian Kelly, co-founder of BreathMasters, Transformational Breathwork elevates the principles of Somatic Release Breathwork by employing targeted mental strategies to influence the subconscious. While Somatic Release might leave some participants feeling unresolved post-session, Transformational Breathwork aims to complete the healing cycle, facilitating a smoother reintegration into everyday life.

This technique not only enhances personal progress through guided mental states but also leverages subconscious reprogramming. By slowing down the brain's frontal cortex—often referred to as the "monkey mind"—it opens a doorway to the subconscious, which is laden with deep-seated beliefs and perceptions that shape our reality. By making the subconscious more accessible, Transformational Breathwork allows for profound shifts and lasting changes, effectively converting what might seem like fate into a conscious choice.

Belief Clearing

A key component of Transformational Breathwork is belief clearing, which actively rewires restrictive thought patterns. In a state of heightened subconscious receptivity achieved during Breathwork sessions, positive affirmations and new beliefs take root much more effectively than in normal waking states. Typically, deep-seated patterns resist change in our usual conscious level, but in the receptive state induced by Breathwork, there's much less resistance to adopting more positive and beneficial belief systems.

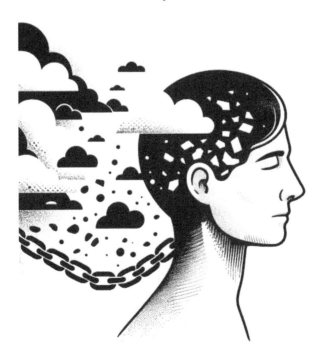

In our everyday conscious state, attempting to think "positive things" can be beneficial, yet often these thoughts don't result in lasting change. This is largely because our subconscious may not be open to new, enhanced thoughts, particularly if they conflict with long-standing patterns established in childhood. However, during Breathwork, our subconscious is more open to new ideas. For example, the belief that we are worthy and deserving of love might be dismissed by our conscious mind as untrue on some level. But in the unique mental state facilitated by Breathwork, our subconscious is more receptive, allowing transformative insights. This receptive state can facilitate life-changing realizations, enabling us to live more authentically.

Transformational Breathwork is versatile, addressing a wide range of human challenges including stress, grief, trauma, anxiety, addiction, depression, chronic pain, fears, phobias, PTSD, relationship issues, and much more. While not everyone experiences immediate transformations, the practice often leads to significant breakthroughs relatively quickly, distinguishing it from other therapeutic treatments. This process of healing is a journey, layer by layer, offering amazing potential for personal growth and transformation.

Healing Deep Wounds with Transformational Breathwork

Trauma has a profound way of embedding itself in our lives, often manifesting in fears and behaviors long after the initial event has passed. One striking example is the story of a woman kidnapped at knifepoint as a child. Tortured and subjected to unthinkable acts, she carried this trauma throughout her life, living in fear and securing her doors each night just to sleep. At 67, she participated in a Transformational 9D Breathwork session led by Brian Kelly, where she managed to envision her captor in a different light and found space in her heart for forgiveness. This pivotal moment allowed her to release the pain and move forward, free from the shackles of her past traumas. Though it may seem extraordinary, such transformative experiences are not uncommon in the realm of Breathwork.

Breathwork teaches us that remembering trauma isn't necessary for healing. Many people carry misconceptions about trauma, believing they must have experienced significant abuse or a

specific traumatic event to justify their feelings. Yet, trauma can be as common as an unattended fall off a bicycle in third grade or even the process of birth itself. The truth is, if you are human, you have experienced some form of trauma.

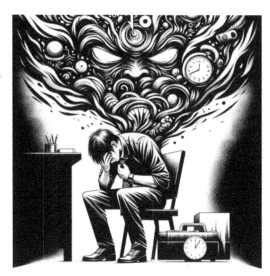

Generational Trauma

Recent studies on how trauma affects families over generations provide further insights by showing us how deeply our ancestors' experiences can influence us. For example in one study, researchers conditioned mice to associate the smell of cherry blossoms with danger causing increased stress. They gave the mice a mild shock while smelling cherry blossoms. This triggered a stress response in the mice that the researchers measured by an increase of the stress hormone cortisol in the mice's blood. Even when the shock wasn't given later on, the mice still felt stressed by the smell. Their cortisol levels would increase just by smelling cherry blossoms even without the shock.

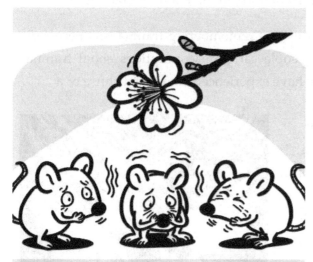

What's amazing is that the mice's babies, who were never shocked, also got stressed by the smell. The original mice's offspring had increased cortisol levels to the smell of cherry blossoms because the DNA passed down had a turned on gene to associate the smell of cherry blossoms with danger regardless of whether the new mice had experienced the same shock stressor. It was not that the parent mice taught their babies to be afraid, the baby mice's DNA did.

Remarkably, the researchers then found that the babies of the babies also had increased stress to the smell despite never having been shocked. More astonishingly still, this stress reaction continued through 14 more generations of mice.

The trauma of the first group of mice was passed down in the DNA from generation to generation. This shows that trauma can be inherited and might explain why we feel stress and anxiety even if we haven't gone through the same things our ancestors did. Think about all the difficult things our ancestors went through—is it any wonder we feel stressed today?!

Addressing and healing our own traumas is crucial, not just for our personal well-being, but also to prevent these burdens from being passed down to future generations. By taking care of and healing our own wounds, we can make sure we don't pass these problems to our children and our children's children. By actively engaging in healing practices like Transformational Breathwork, we help ourselves move past old traumas while also halting this cycle of transmission. We can not only free ourselves but also help ensure that subsequent generations can lead healthier and happier lives without these hardships.

Transformational Breathwork offers a powerful way to release deep-rooted trauma. It helps our bodies understand that past dangers are over, allowing us to work through and let go of built-up emotional energy. Through this practice, we can face and heal from old traumas, freeing ourselves from their long-lasting effects and leading a life that is more free and true to who we are.

Harnessing the Theta Brainwave State in Transformational Breathwork

Transformational Breathwork effectively guides us into the Theta brainwave state, a deeply restorative and hypnotic state of awareness. By intentionally entering this state, we step away from the incessant chatter of our "monkey minds" and tap into our subconscious operating system. Here, our receptivity to suggestions and openness to new ideas are greatly enhanced.

From the age of two until eight years old, we lived mostly in the Theta brainwave state. During this period, our prefrontal cortex was not fully developed, meaning we operated on feelings rather than analytical thought. In this state of natural hypnosis, we absorbed everything from our environment without the ability to critically assess it. This is why young children are so impressionable, soaking up behaviors, beliefs, and emotions from those around them. Good or bad, all these experiences become deeply ingrained in our subconscious.

Once we reach adulthood, accessing the Theta state through Transformational Breathwork provides an opportunity to revisit and reprogram these early, deeply embedded patterns. The Theta brainwave state is akin to the natural hypnosis we experience right upon waking and just before sleeping, times when our minds are particularly receptive. This is why home hypnosis courses often recommend practice during these periods.

Through Transformational Breathwork, we can profoundly shift our perspectives. With the right guidance, it's possible to reframe challenges and struggles, viewing them through a new lens. This shift allows us to realize that the true issue often isn't the problem itself, but our relationship to it. By changing this relationship, what were once perceived as problems transform into opportunities for growth and deeper self-awareness.

This state is not just about temporary relief; it's about making lasting changes in how we perceive and interact with our world. The Theta brainwave state accessed during Transformational Breathwork provides a unique opportunity for deep, lasting, transformative healing, allowing us to rewrite old narratives and embrace a more empowered way of living.

Breathing Through the Mouth with Intention

In a previous chapter, we emphasized the benefits of nasal breathing over mouth breathing and discussed how excessive loss of CO_2 can pose issues for the body. It might seem contradictory, then, that a powerful Breathwork technique like

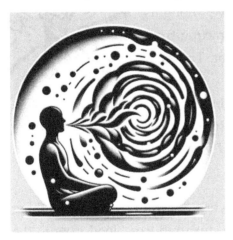

Somatic Release and Transformational Breathwork involves intense mouth breathing and the resultant lower CO_2 levels. However, there is a purposeful distinction: this method involves relatively short, deliberate periods of mouth breathing as a therapeutic tool.

This approach is designed to bypass the conscious mind, which often blocks the reframing of deep-seated, limiting beliefs held in our subconscious. To access and alter these ingrained patterns, we need to quiet the conscious thinking mind and enter a specific mental state known as the Theta brainwave state. While we naturally visit this state every morning as we are waking up and each night before sleep, achieving it while awake through meditation is challenging for most, especially amidst the distractions of modern life. Somatic Release and Transformational Breathwork offers a shortcut to this state.

After engaging in mouth breathing at an increased rate for about 10 to 15 minutes, we achieve transient hypofrontality. Let's unpack this phrase: "Transient" implies a temporary state; we are not altering our brain function permanently but rather momentarily in order to facilitate healing. "Hypo" indicates reduction, and "frontality" refers to the activity in the prefrontal cortex, the region of the brain responsible for conscious analysis and planning.

The prefrontal cortex which is crucial for what makes us uniquely human, can also trap us in loops of obsessive thoughts about the past and future, detracting from our ability to live in the present. Transient hypofrontality, therefore, involves 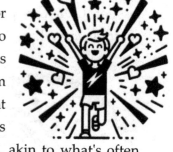 temporarily reducing activity in this area, akin to what's often described as "Flow State" or "Runner's High." It's a state where brain activity slows down, and we perform optimally, focused entirely on the present.

During these types of Breathwork, the rapid mouth breathing decreases CO_2 levels, which in turn reduces blood flow to the prefrontal cortex. This decrease in CO_2 constricts the 60,000+ miles of blood vessels in our body, effectively "cutting off" the fuel to our overactive minds. This is when the profound shifts occur—when mental activity slows, the chattering mind steps back, and the usual boundaries between self and surroundings begin to dissolve.

When we suddenly experience our problems are not as overwhelming as they previously seemed—this is the moment we bypass the analytical mind, allowing ourselves to be free from limiting beliefs and patterns, even if just temporarily. This mental relaxation can lead to feelings of euphoria or transcendence, often described as a "spiritual experience."

Imagine our brain as a bank vault that we have just unlocked. This state grants access to repressed memories and experiences, providing a unique opportunity to process and integrate what has been buried. With the "monkey mind" out of the way, we can transcend our narrow self-views and feel deeply connected to everything around us. Experiencing this interconnectedness can be transformative, making it nearly impossible to see ourselves as limited or insignificant ever again. This is the profound potential of breathing through the mouth with a purpose.

What Happens in a Transformational Breathwork Journey?

Every Transformational Breathwork session is unique, not just across individuals but also from one session to the next. Every time we breathe, we learn something new. A testament to this variability is a man who has participated in Brian Kelly's signature 9D Breathwork journey 67 times, with each experience differing from the last. What needs to come up will surface when the time is right, reflecting our ongoing growth and changes. Each session is an opportunity to peel away another layer of the onion in our healing journey. This variability reflects our personal growth and shifting internal landscapes; as we evolve, the barriers that once held us back change, revealing new layers of our emotional and spiritual selves to explore and heal.

During a Transformational Breathwork journey or any of the other conscious connected breathing Breathwork methods, participants may encounter a range of profound experiences. Most of the time Breathwork is energizing. If you feel depleted going in, you might feel activated going out.

Some report spiritual awakenings, feeling an intense connection to something greater than themselves or transcending time and space. This often manifests as profound sensations of love, joy, bliss, kindness, oneness, and a sense of purpose and meaning.

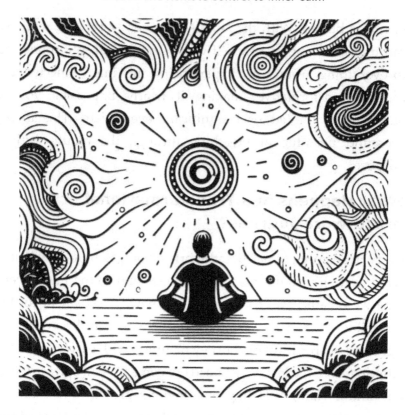

Others experience cathartic releases, where the technique of conscious connected breathing facilitates the physical release of repressed and suppressed emotions that have been locked within the body. It's not uncommon for participants to simply fall asleep, which is just as valid and necessary for those individuals. For some, a Breathwork session will be the only time during a busy week when they can have time to truly rest. The body takes what it needs from the session.

In these journeys, there is no incorrect way to respond. The key is to enter the experience without judgment and allow whatever needs to surface to do so. Each Breathwork session is a step along the continuous path of personal transformation and healing, providing whatever the participant needs at that moment in their life.

Potential Experiences During Somatic Release or Transformational Breathwork

As we embark on our Somatic Release or Transformational Breathwork journey, it's important to approach the experience with an open mind and a willingness to embrace whatever arises. Whether we encounter intense physical sensations, emotional releases, or mental resistance, each response is a valuable part of the healing process. Uncomfortable feelings or sensations may surface to be released from the body, and that is what we want. Understanding these potential experiences prepares us to navigate them with confidence and compassion for ourselves. Remember, the goal is not to control or judge what comes up, but to allow the breath to guide us through a profound process of self-discovery and transformation.

Physical Sensations

In these types of Breathwork, deep breathing can lead to various physical sensations as a result of the quick exchange of oxygen and carbon dioxide. These sensations are normal and not a cause for concern. You might experience tightness, numbness or tingling in your fingertips, toes, or lips. Sometimes, your hands might cramp up, creating what is known as "tetany" or "lobster claws" or "T-rex hands," where

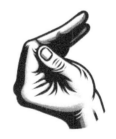

your fingers jam together in a five digit point and you feel unable to move them temporarily. Don't worry—you won't get stuck like that. This is normal. It is a common response and will subside once you stop the intense breathing. Breathe and focus on relaxing the muscles between the shoulder blades. Often, these physical sensations precede significant emotional releases if you can ride through them to allow the release. Remember, you are safe and in control. You are just breathing. You can always slow your breathing if needed. Whether you choose to push through and face your dragon today or slow it down for now, trust the process and be kind to yourself.

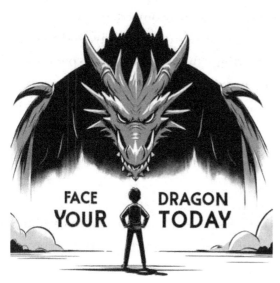

During breathing, areas of the body you didn't even realize were tight might suddenly release. It can wake up areas of the body you didn't know were fast asleep. Breathing can actually decrease pain as the breath can send a rush of pain-killing endorphins to the whole body. You may feel the need to move or shake your arms or legs. The body has its own knowledge. Breathe into it. And listen.

Sometimes, you might feel discomfort in different parts of the body during Breathwork. This can manifest in the arms, legs, neck, or chest—often where we hold a lot of tension, now exposed by the breath. While the rest of your body is opening up, these muscles might be clinging tightly. Try to relax the area while mentally sending your breath to where the tension is. Breathe into the discomfort. You can also apply firm pressure to the tense area while breathing deeply into your fingertips. This may result in a deep physical release—often accompanied by an emotional release.

You may experience major fluctuations in temperature during a session. You may feel cold at one point but then break into a sweat as energy starts moving through your body.

After releasing trapped emotions, you might momentarily forget to breathe. This is also totally normal. When you realize this, simply return to the breathing technique and continue. Start again. You released one layer of the onion and there are more layers to peel away. Whatever happens in the body, just breathe into it and through it. There is nothing to worry about. Trust the process. You are safe. If you want to go deep, breathe deep.

Emotional Releases

Emotions are likely to surface during these types of Breathwork, and this is a key part of the healing process. If emotions don't come up, it may be that your journey is focused more on the physical aspects this time, but healing is still taking place. When emotions do rise, it's crucial not to suppress them. Let them come up and out. Feel them and release them. Despite what your mind may tell you, emotions cannot kill you. Feeling emotions is safe and essential for healing. If you need to cry, scream, shake, or laugh, allow yourself to do so. These expressions are ways of releasing pent-up energy from unprocessed emotions and trapped trauma. Pushing emotions down halts your healing, so let them flow freely. It is natural for one emotion to lead to another; for instance, anger might be followed by sadness. After an emotional release, return to the breathing technique to continue processing unprocessed emotions. Keep peeling those layers back.

Mental Challenges

In the initial 10 to 15 minutes of the Breathwork journey, your mind might resist and try to distract you. After the first 15 minutes, the mind will calm down and enjoy the ride, but in the beginning, it will fight you. It may tell you that the practice is too difficult, pointless, or that you should stop for various reasons. This resistance is natural as your mind is accustomed to a state of chronic stress, and it fears change. The mind wants to keep you stuck, but choosing to do these types of Breathwork means you have made a different choice. You have chosen healing. When distractions arise, refocus on your breath. Imagine your mind as a dog on a leash—when it strays, gently bring it back on track. By choosing to engage fully in the practice, you are committing to your healing journey.

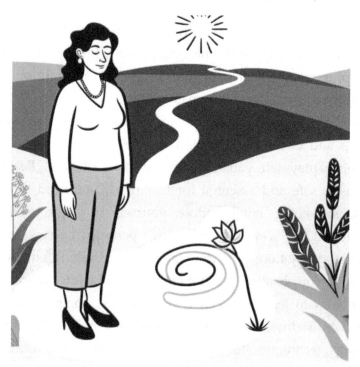

Mastering the Technique for Transformational Breathwork

Now that we've discussed what to expect physically, emotionally, and mentally during a Somatic Release or Transformational Breathwork journey, let's delve into the specific breathing technique used in Transformational Breathwork to navigate this transformative experience. The most common method used is known as the "Two-Part Belly Breath." This technique is straightforward, so let's try it out:

1. Position Your Hands:
Place your right hand on your chest and your left hand on your belly.

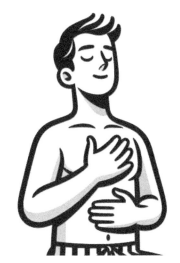

2. Breathe into Your Belly:
Inhale deeply so that your left hand rises first as your belly expands.

3. Breathe into Your Chest: Continue the same breath up into your chest, feeling your right hand rise.

4. Relax and Release: Exhale, relax, and let the air flow out naturally—no need to force it.

Give it a try: Inhale into the belly, then the chest, and relax to exhale. If your hands aren't moving much, try to deepen your breaths—remember, it's more important to breathe deeply than quickly. This belly-chest pattern should create a wave-like motion in your breathing. Start gently, and you can increase the intensity as you get comfortable.

The Role of Music and Setting

As you practice these types of Breathwork, the accompanying music will guide your journey. It starts slow, intensifies in the middle, and then slows down towards the end. This progression mirrors the emotional and physical release you might experience. Feel free to adjust your breathing pace—speed up to intensify the release or slow down if it becomes too much. The key is to keep breathing deeply, regardless of the pace.

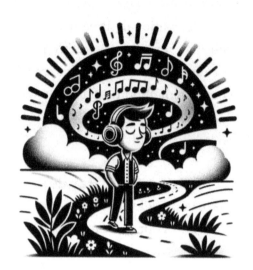

Preparing for Any Breathwork Session

Before beginning, make sure you are fully prepared:

- **Position:** Lie down in a comfortable position without a pillow under your head to avoid restricting your breathing. A rolled up towel under the neck can be used if that feels more comfortable. Some people are prone to coughing spells and benefit from having the head slightly elevated in a reclined recliner.

- **Environment:** Ensure a quiet, undisturbed space. Keep pets and children in another room if possible. This time is for you.

- **Accessories:** Have a blanket for warmth, water, lip balm if needed, and a pillow—not for your head, but to muffle any screams if you feel the need to release loudly without disturbing others.

You Cannot Mess This Up

Remember, there's no wrong way to do this. When in a Transformational Breathwork session, if you find yourself getting caught up mentally in the Two-Part Belly Breath technique, simply focus on deep belly breaths. Breathe deep into your belly so your abdomen goes up and down. If you are thinking about the technique, then you are thinking and not feeling. Deep breaths into the belly will still get you there, it simply may take longer. I often switch back and forth depending on what feels right for me in the moment. The goal of these types of Breathwork is to release stress, not create more of it. You already know how to breathe; trust in that. Use this time to address the chronic stress that has impacted your life for years. Imagine releasing years of pent-up emotion in just over one hour, breath by breath, and emerging with a newfound peace. It is worth it.

Assessing the Risks of Somatic Release and Transformational Breathwork

While Breathwork is considered one of the safest healing modalities—safer than many medications prescribed today—there are certain contraindications and precautions to be aware of. Unlike other practices, the most serious adverse events linked to Breathwork have occurred underwater, making land-based sessions significantly safer. However, if there are any potential concerns, consulting with a physician first is advised. A useful guideline is: "When in doubt—sit it out."

Listed Contraindications:

Seizure Disorders: Rapid breathing can potentially trigger seizures.

Pregnancy: Particularly in the third trimester, intense Breathwork could induce preterm labor. When pregnant, it is best to wait until pregnancy is over to try Somatic Release or Transformational Breathwork. Try a more restorative breathing method instead with gentle, controlled nasal breathing and cease immediately if discomfort occurs..

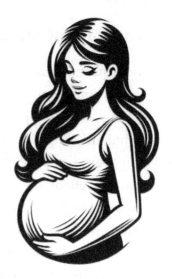

Cardiovascular Disease:
Individuals with
 conditions such as coronary artery disease, abnormal heart rhythms, aneurysms, uncontrolled blood pressure, recent heart attacks, or other heart-related issues should exercise caution. Relaxation-focused Breathwork might be more suitable, or modifications like nasal breathing could be safer alternatives.

Severe Pulmonary Disease: Conditions like COPD, asthma, and lung cancer require caution. Asthmatic participants should have a rescue inhaler handy and consult a doctor before participating.

Severe Psychiatric Disorders: Disorders like schizophrenia or severe bipolar disorder are listed as contraindications, so consultation with a physician is advisable. However, studies show no adverse reactions and that Breathwork may be beneficial for these conditions.

Recent Surgery: Post-surgical patients should allow wounds to heal for at least three months before attempting intense Breathwork.

These types of Breathwork induce a purposeful sympathetic state, which could theoretically strain the heart, hence the contraindications. Gentler Breathwork with nasal breathing that promotes a parasympathetic state may be universally safer.

Research and Safety

A significant study on Holotropic Breathwork—a method involving 3 hours of connected conscious breathing compared to the 30-45 minutes of intense breathing with Somatic Release and Transformational Breathwork—showed no adverse reactions among 11,000 psychiatric inpatients over 12 years. This underscores the low-risk nature of Breathwork, even in its more intense forms. Breathwork is a low risk therapy.

Addressing Common Concerns:

One concern is the potential for re-traumatization. However, as long as Breathwork is conducted in a safe setting (not underwater) and with proper guidance, the risk is minimal. Fainting is a possibility, which is why Somatic Release and Transformational Breathwork sessions are typically conducted in a lying or reclined position. This safe posture allows participants to experience potentially profound visions or spiritual insights without risk. The biggest challenge is having uncomfortable emotions stirred up which is a great opportunity for healing, learning, and growth. Some ideas for supportive aftercare to complement the session and help with any residual emotions include a walk in nature, time with a supportive friend, a therapy session, or a bike ride.

Always remember that you control the intensity of your Breathwork. You can choose to breathe faster or slow down and breathe through your nose. Listening to your body is crucial; if you feel panicky, simply slow your breathing. Despite fears to the contrary, emotions themselves are not harmful—it is safe to feel.

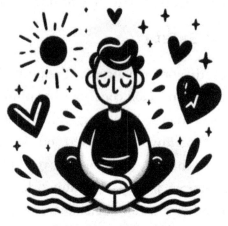

IT IS SAFE TO FEEL.

Brian Kelly has safely conducted Transformational Breathwork for over 20,000 students without serious incidents, confirming its status as a low-risk therapy. The key is to stay mindful and responsive to our body's signals throughout the experience. If you ever feel the need to deepen the experience, remember that deeper breathing should be approached with attentiveness to your physical and emotional responses.

After the Journey: Navigating Post-Breathwork

Somatic Release and Transformational Breathwork sessions can be profound, often leaving participants with a wide array of sensations and emotions. As we emerge from these deeply personal journeys, it's important to understand that what we experience can vary greatly from one session to another. Let's discuss the diverse experiences one might encounter, from the immediate aftermath to the days following a Breathwork session, and offer practical aftercare advice to support the integration process.

Different Experiences Within Journeys

These types of Breathwork can lead to a wide range of experiences, each unique to the individual. These might include:

Emotional Release: Feelings of joy, fear, hurt, sadness, anger, or relief as pent-up emotions are processed.

Physical Sensations: Tingling, lightness, or heaviness as energy moves through the body. Any muscle cramps may suggest a deficiency in magnesium which can be bought as an over-the-counter supplement taken at night.

Mental Clarity: Moments of insight or profound realizations about personal life or patterns.

Spiritual Connection: A sense of unity, connection to something greater, or spiritual awakening.

After the Session:

-**Emotional Integration:** You may feel a sense of emotional release with amazing happiness, filled with energy and power or your experience may be one of shock or overwhelm by the emotions that surfaced. Whatever you experience, do not judge and be kind to you. Gradually process and integrate the emotions and insights gained during the session.

Physical Changes: Feelings of lightness or heaviness, tingling, or a general sense of bodily awareness. Increased body awareness, potential shifts in posture or breathing patterns.

Mental and Spiritual Growth: Enhanced clarity or new perspectives on personal issues. Development of new mental frameworks, deepened self-awareness, and spiritual insights.

Aftercare Practices

After a Breathwork session, it's common to experience a wide range of sensations. You might feel super energized, or you could feel depleted, raw, and windblown in the first hour or even a day or two afterwards. It's crucial to take care of yourself during this time to help your body and mind recover and integrate the session's experiences.

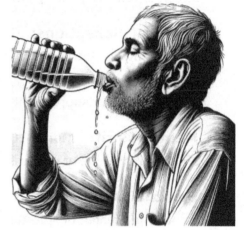

Hydration: Water is essential to help flush out toxins released during the Breathwork session. Make sure to drink plenty of water to stay hydrated.

Be Sweet to Yourself: If you feel tender or vulnerable, treat yourself with kindness. Engage in activities that nurture your body and soul.

Rest: Ensure you get enough rest to allow your body and mind to recover and integrate the session's experiences.

Stretching: Gentle stretching can help release any residual tension in your body and promote relaxation.

Grounding Practices: Walking barefoot on grass, spending time in nature, or engaging in gentle movement can help you feel more grounded.

Journaling: Write down your experiences, feelings, and any insights gained during the session. This can help you process and integrate your journey.

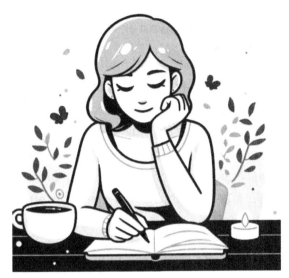

Talking: Share your experience with a trusted friend, therapist, or support group if you feel comfortable.

Check-in with Yourself: Regularly assess how you're feeling physically, emotionally, and mentally. Notice any shifts or changes that have occurred since your Breathwork session.

Seek Support: If you find it challenging to integrate your experiences, feel overwhelmed or want to explore the next level of intentional integration consider seeking professional support.

Embracing the Journey

Engaging in Somatic Release and Transformational Breathwork is a profound way to address and release physical, emotional, and mental blockages. Each journey is a step towards deeper healing and self-awareness. By embracing whatever arises with an open heart and mind, you can experience transformative and revitalizing changes that enrich and better your life. Check out TheBreathMD.com for opportunities to experience this amazing healing experience for yourself.

Transformational Breathwork - Shifting Beliefs and Unlocking Inner Healing

More purposely and effectively than Somatic Release Breathwork which capably facilitates the release of trapped emotions, Transformational Breathwork also aids in letting go of old habits and shifting deeply ingrained belief structures. Remarkably, both processes bypass the need for verbalizing issues, making them a powerful alternative to talk therapy. While talk therapy has its merits, it often requires articulating feelings or identifying problems, which can be challenging.

These types of Breathwork, on the other hand, cut directly to the root of issues causing lifelong struggles such as anxiety, stress, poor sleep, low energy, self-worth issues, and various mental complexities. They often work without needing to pinpoint the exact problem, offering a fast track to profound healing and personal transformation. By harnessing the power of the breath, these techniques bring suppressed emotions to the surface, enabling the release of negative thought patterns, limiting beliefs, and self-sabotage behaviors. Many people experience life-changing breakthroughs after just one session, finding relief from treatment-resistant depression and other persistent issues.

The core strength of Transformational Breathwork lies in its ability to penetrate the subconscious swiftly and process deep-seated traumas and emotions. Unlike other methods that rely solely on the breath, Transformational Breathwork combines Breathwork with verbal guidance and coaching, navigating individuals to release limiting beliefs and dysfunctional patterns when the subconscious is most receptive. This dual approach not only utilizes the breath as medicine but also incorporates targeted coaching to help release suppressed emotions, childhood traumas, and generational burdens. It opens a powerful gateway to the depths of the psyche, offering access to profound healing and transformation that might otherwise remain unreachable.

Deep Breaths, Deeper Healing: The Power of Somatic and Transformational Breathwork

Somatic Release and Transformational Breathwork are exceptional practices that promise the potential for profound personal transformation. Both practices utilize the powerful technique of circular connected breathing to help restoring the vital

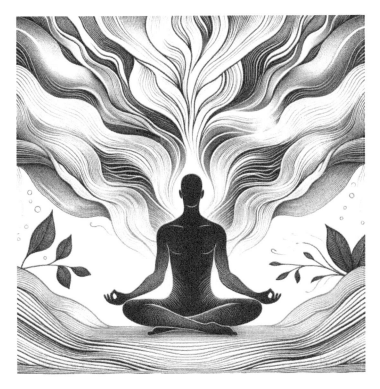

connection between the mind and the body's wisdom. By engaging in these breathing techniques, you can explore deep layers of the self, releasing burdens of the past and embracing a renewed sense of presence and vitality.

If you're seeking a method to navigate and transform the stresses and emotional weights of daily life, Somatic Release and Transformational Breathwork offer compelling avenues. They don't just address the symptoms but dive deep into the cause, allowing for a realignment of emotional and physical states. As tools for healing, learning, and growth, these Breathwork practices stand out as profound aids in the journey toward holistic well-being. Embrace the opportunity to transform; explore these powerful practices and witness the substantial benefits in your own life.

7
THE ART OF BREATH: EXPLORING TECHNIQUES FOR WELLNESS

"Your breath is your greatest ally in the journey of healing. Trust in its rhythm, and it will guide you back to wholeness."

- Emily Maroutian

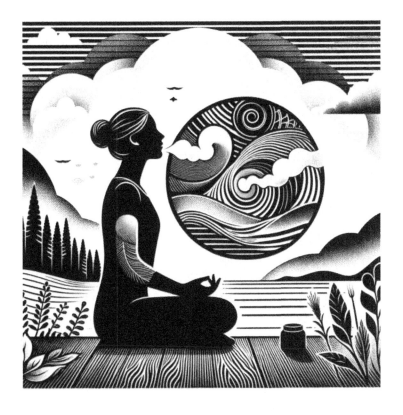

When Breathing Becomes Breathwork

Breathing transforms into Breathwork when we bring focused attention and intention to the process. Whether we are breathing in a specific pattern, breathing powerfully and intensely for a preset period of time, or slowing down our breath 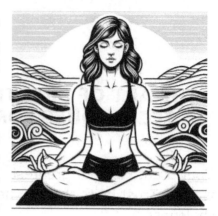 during cardiovascular training, these are all forms of Breathwork. If we already have a regular meditation routine or yoga practice, we are likely engaging in a form of Breathwork as well. This chapter will delve into various Breathwork techniques, offering a diverse array of practices to help us harness the power of our breath. From diaphragmatic breathing to pranayama, mindful breathing to breath visualization, each technique provides unique benefits and applications, enhancing our physical, mental, and emotional well-being. Let's explore how these practices can transform our breath into a powerful tool for health and vitality.

Breathwork Techniques

In many ancient traditions, people believed that our breath carried life energy through our bodies. By understanding and using our breath, we can tap into this energy and improve our overall well-being. There are many types of Breathwork, each with unique benefits. Each method could have an entire book written on it—in fact, most of them do. Some methods work better for some people, while others are drawn to different types of breathing. My intention is to give you a sampling of the many beneficial types of Breathwork available. Most of these breath techniques are focused on more long-term chronic stress relief that you can incorporate into your daily journey. As with anything in life, try out various types of Breathwork and see what resonates with you. Experiment to discover what works best for your body and mind.

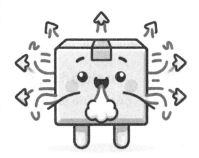

Before we dive into new techniques, let's revisit some of the Breathwork methods we've already explored. You may remember The Box Breath which is actually a Pranayama technique from Chapter 1, a simple yet powerful method to calm the mind. In Chapter 4, we discussed Heart Coherence Breathing, which helps synchronize your heart and brain for enhanced emotional regulation. Chapter 6 introduced several transformative practices, including Circular Connected Breathing used in Transformational Breathwork, Somatic Release Breathwork, and the Two-part Belly Breath. Each of these techniques offers unique benefits and can serve as a foundation for exploring the new methods in this chapter.

Diaphragmatic Breathing: The Foundation of Calm

Over the past few decades, scientists have conducted numerous studies exploring the effects of Breathwork on stress reduction and health. The results have been overwhelmingly positive, providing strong evidence for the effectiveness of Breathwork promoting relaxation, reducing stress, and improving overall well-being.

One of the most well studied forms of Breathwork is diaphragmatic breathing, also known as deep belly breathing. This involves breathing deeply to the diaphragm, allowing the abdomen to rise and fall with each breath. Research has shown that diaphragmatic breathing can activate the parasympathetic nervous system, leading to reductions in heart rate, blood pressure, and the stress hormone cortisol. Here's how to practice diaphragmatic breathing:

1.   **Position:** Sit or lie down in a comfortable position, with your spine straight and your shoulders relaxed.

2.   **Hand Placement:** Place one hand on your chest and the other hand on your abdomen. This will help you become aware of the movement of your breath.

3.   **Inhale:** As you inhale deeply through your nose, imagine filling your abdomen with air like a balloon. Feel your abdomen rise as it expands with each breath.

4.   **Exhale**: As you exhale slowly through your mouth, feel your abdomen gently deflate as you release the air.

5.   **Repeat for Several Breaths:** Continue to breathe deeply and slowly, focusing on the sensation of your abdomen rising and falling with each breath.

Diaphragmatic breathing is a powerful tool for reducing stress and promoting relaxation. By engaging the diaphragm and taking slow, deep breaths, we can activate the body's relaxation response, triggering the release of feel-good hormones like serotonin and endorphins. This can help lower blood pressure, reduce muscle tension, and promote a sense of calmness and well-being.

4-4-6 Breathing Pattern

The 4-4-6 breathing pattern is a controlled breathing exercise designed to promote relaxation, reduce stress, and improve overall respiratory function. It is one of my favorites and is what I typically use as my 90-second remote control to inner calm. This technique involves a specific sequence of inhaling, holding the breath, and exhaling. The steps to perform this technique are as follows:

1. Inhale: Breathe in slowly and deeply through your nose for a count of 4 seconds.

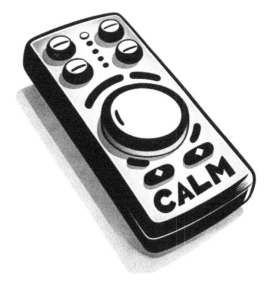

2. Hold: Hold your breath for a count of 4 seconds.

3. Exhale: Exhale slowly and completely through your mouth or nose for a count of 6 seconds (or however long until you empty your lungs).

Do not get hung up on the counts. This is to decrease stress—not increase it. It is all about the ratio. As long as the total time inhaling is less than the total time not inhaling, you are activating calming in your body.

The benefits of the 4-4-6 breathing pattern include reducing stress and anxiety by activating the parasympathetic nervous system, enhancing focus and mental clarity, and improving respiratory efficiency. Additionally, it promotes better sleep by calming the mind and preparing the body for rest, and supports emotional regulation by helping individuals manage their emotional responses. This technique can be incorporated into daily routines to maintain a state of calm and balance, used during stressful situations to regain composure, improve respiratory function, and employed as part of a pre-sleep routine to ease the transition into sleep.

Pursed Lip Breathing

Pursed lip breathing is a simple yet effective technique used to control shortness of breath and enhance oxygenation, making it especially beneficial for individuals with chronic obstructive pulmonary disease (COPD), asthma, or other respiratory conditions. The technique involves relaxing the neck and shoulder muscles, inhaling slowly through the nose for about two to four counts while keeping the mouth closed, then pursing the lips as if to whistle or gently blow out a candle, and exhaling slowly through the pursed lips for about four to eight counts, taking twice as long to exhale as to inhale. It is all about the ratio. 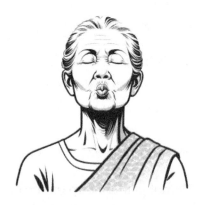 Purposely making the exhale longer than the inhale sends a signal to your heart that tells your brain that everything is ok—no danger here. Don't get hung up on the exact numbers—whether you are counting correctly or doing it right (you don't even have to purse your lips if it would be awkward in a public setting)—simply make the exhale longer than the inhale. This simple adjustment of the inhale-exhale ratio immediately shifts the body to a calmer state.

The mechanism behind pursed lip breathing involves creating slight back pressure in the airways during exhalation, which helps keep the small airways in the lungs open and prevents air trapping, allowing for more efficient gas exchange. It also makes it easier to extend the exhale through pursed lips. Clinically, it is commonly recommended as part of pulmonary rehabilitation for COPD patients and can help manage asthma symptoms by reducing the work of breathing. Additionally, it serves as a valuable relaxation technique to manage stress and anxiety.

Pursed lip breathing is a practical tool for anyone experiencing difficulty breathing. It offers immediate relief and long-term benefits when practiced regularly, making it a vital component of respiratory health management.

Pranayama: Ancient Breathing Practices for Modern Life

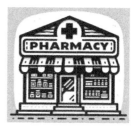

Pranayama, which translates to "control of life force" in Sanskrit, refers to a set of ancient breathing techniques developed in the yogic tradition of India. These practices are designed to harness the power of the breath to balance the body and mind, promote health and vitality, and awaken spiritual awareness. Pranayama has been described as the pharmacy of breath—for almost any ailment, there is a breath technique to fix it. Here are some common pranayama techniques:

1. Alternate Nostril Breathing (Nadi Shodhana):
This technique involves alternating the flow of breath between the left and right nostrils using the fingers to block one nostril at a time. It is believed to balance the energy channels in the body and promote a sense of calm and balance.

2. Skull-Shining Breath (Kapalabhati): This technique involves rapid, forceful exhalations followed by passive inhalations. It is thought to cleanse the respiratory system, increase energy levels, and improve mental clarity.

3. Bee Breath (Bhramari): This technique involves inhaling deeply and then exhaling while making a humming sound like a bee which also increases your nitric oxide levels known to improve oxygen delivery to your brain and body. It is believed to calm the mind, reduce anxiety, and promote inner peace.

4. Victorious Breath (Ujjayi): This technique involves breathing in and out through the nose while slightly constricting the back of the throat to create a sound like ocean waves. It is thought to increase oxygenation, improve concentration,

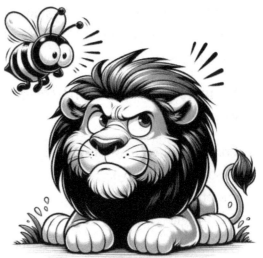

and induce a state of deep relaxation.

5. Lion's Breath (Simhasana): This technique is designed to release tension and anger while stimulating the throat and chest. The practice involves inhaling deeply through the nose, and then exhaling forcefully with the mouth open wide, tongue extended, and making a roaring sound like a lion. It reduces stress, improves circulation, clears the respiratory tract, and promotes a sense of empowerment by energetically releasing pent-up emotions and tension.

Pranayama practices can be a powerful addition to our Breathwork toolkit, offering a variety of techniques to support our physical, mental, and spiritual well-being. Videos depicting many of the techniques can be found on TheBreathMD.com. Whether we are looking to reduce stress, increase energy, or deepen our spiritual practice, there's a pranayama technique for us.

Mindful Breathing: Bringing Awareness to the Present Moment

Mindful breathing is another area of research interest, with studies suggesting that mindfulness-based breathing practices can help reduce symptoms of depression, anxiety, and post-traumatic stress disorder (PTSD). By bringing awareness to the present moment and focusing on the sensations of the breath, mindful breathing can help quiet the mind and promote a sense of calm and relaxation. It is a simple yet powerful practice that can help us cultivate present-moment awareness.

Mindful breathing is a form of meditation that involves bringing focused attention to the breath and the sensations associated with breathing. Taking a breath with consciousness turns the automatic into something intentional. We will take millions of breaths in a lifetime. But what about this one? Will it be nothing more than the breath between the last one and the next one? Or will we empower it with something more? We can take a breath. Take the next one like our life depends on it. Because it does.

Here's how to practice mindful breathing:

1. Position: Sit or lie down in a comfortable position, with your spine straight and your shoulders relaxed.

2.   Close Your Eyes (optional): If it feels comfortable for you, gently close your eyes to help minimize distractions.

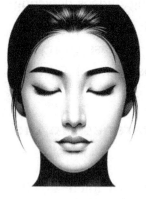

3.   Attention: Bring you attention to your breath. Begin by simply observing your breath as it enters and leaves your body. Notice the sensation of the air moving in and out of your nostrils, the rise and fall of your chest or abdomen, and any other sensations associated with breathing.

4.   Focus On the Present Moment: As you continue to breathe mindfully, notice any thoughts, feelings, or sensations that arise without judgment. If your mind starts to wander, gently bring your attention back to your breath.

5.   Practice Non-Reactivity: Allow your breath to be an anchor for your awareness, bringing you back to the present moment whenever you find yourself getting caught up in thoughts or emotions.

Mindful breathing can be practiced anywhere, anytime, and for any length of time. Whether we have just a few minutes or a longer period of time to dedicate to the practice, even a few moments of mindful breathing can have profound benefits for our mental and emotional well-being.

Visualization and Breathwork: Harnessing the Power of the Mind-Body Connection

Visualization is a technique that involves using mental imagery to create a sense of relaxation, and calmness. When combined with Breathwork, visualization can be a powerful tool for reducing stress, enhancing performance, and promoting healing.

Here's how to practice visualization and Breathwork:

1. Position: Sit or lie down in a comfortable position in a quiet, comfortable space, with your spine straight and your shoulders relaxed.

2. Calm Yourself: Close your eyes and take a few deep breaths to help relax your body and calm your mind.

3. Positive Scene: Choose a positive image or scenario. Choose a mental image or scenario that evokes feelings of relaxation, calmness, and well-being. This could be a peaceful beach, a tranquil forest, or a favorite vacation spot.

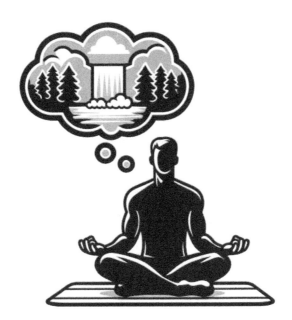

4. Be There: Imagine yourself in the scene. Close your eyes and imagine yourself in the chosen image or scenario. Use all of your senses to make the visualization as vivid and realistic as possible. Notice the sights, sounds, smells, and sensations associated with the scene.

5.   Breathe Deeply and Slowly: As you continue to visualize, focus on taking slow, deep breaths. Allow your breath to deepen your sense of relaxation and connection to the visualization.

Visualization and Breathwork can be a powerful combination for reducing stress and promoting relaxation. By using the power of our imagination and our breath, we can create a sense of calmness and well-being that can help us cope with stress and navigate life's challenges more effectively. Whether we are dealing with everyday stressors or facing a specific challenge, visualization and Breathwork can provide a valuable tool for promoting health and well-being.

4-7-8 Breathing: A Simple Technique for Quick Relaxation

The 4-7-8 breathing technique, popularized by Dr. Andrew Weil, is a simple yet powerful practice for achieving deep relaxation and reducing stress. This method involves a specific breathing pattern designed to calm the nervous system. Here's how to practice 4-7-8 breathing:

1. Sit or Lie Down: Find a comfortable position.

2. Position the Tongue: Place the tip of your tongue against the ridge of tissue just behind your upper front teeth and keep it there throughout the practice.

3. Exhale Completely Through the Mouth: You can optionally add a whooshing sound.

4. Inhale Through the Nose: Close your mouth and inhale quietly through your nose to a mental count of four.

5. Breath Hold: Hold your breath for a count of seven.

6. Exhale Through the Mouth: Exhale completely through your mouth to a count of eight. If you do not have enough air for the entire 8 count, simply hold on the exhale until you reach 8. Do not stress about the numbers or whether you are "doing it right" because the point is to calm down and relax—not get hung up on the technique.

7. Repeat: This completes one breath. Now inhale again and repeat the cycle.

The 4-7-8 breathing technique is a quick and effective way to calm the mind, reduce anxiety, and prepare for sleep. Regular practice can help us manage stress more effectively and improve overall well-being.

Wim Hof Method: Breathing for Resilience

This method, developed by Wim Hof, also known as "The Iceman," is a powerful technique that combines specific breathing techniques, cold exposure, and unwavering commitment to improve health and well-being. His remarkable feats include climbing Everest in shorts, running a marathon in the Namib Desert without water, and submerging himself in ice for a record-breaking one hour, 52 minutes, and 42 seconds. Known for his infectious charisma, Hof's mission is to bring "strength, happiness, and health" to people worldwide.

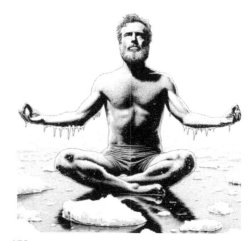

Wim Hof's approach is encapsulated in his mantra, "feeling is understanding." The breathing component of the Wim Hof Method involves controlled hyperventilation (often called "superventilation" in the Breathwork world as it is done on purpose and produces outstanding results) followed by breath retention. The Wim Hof Method diverges from other breathing modalities due to the presence of prolonged breath holds (retentions) and its efficiency (lasting results in just 15 minutes a day). Here's how to practice the basic breathing technique:

1. Preparation: Sit or lie down in a comfortable, safe space. If sitting, ensure there are no hard objects nearby to avoid injury if you feel lightheaded. Lying down is preferable for safety. Close your eyes clearing your mind. Remember to listen to your body as it gives you signals for use as personal feedback to modify the practice to work best for you.

2. Deep Breaths: Take 30 deep breaths. Inhale deeply through your nose or mouth, filling your lungs completely, allowing the air to fill up your belly, your chest, and all the way up to your head. Exhale through your mouth, releasing the air but not forcefully. Continue this cycle rapidly, aiming to feel slightly lightheaded or experience tingling sensations. Focus on "energizing" with each inhale and "letting go" with each exhale.

3. Breath Retention: After the 30th exhale, draw in one more big breath filling your lungs to maximum capacity without using any force, then relax to let all the air out. Hold your breath with your lungs empty. Hold until you feel a strong urge to breathe again—and then hold a little longer. It is not mandatory but you can time yourself with a stopwatch. Relax your entire body and see how long you can go without breathing. Success lies in how much you can relax all your muscles while holding no air in your lungs. This is an act of will. Remember, your oxygen level is just fine—CO_2 levels are what make you feel air hunger. This technique can show you how much power you have to control your body as well as your stress and anxiety. As you get happier, healthier, and stronger, you'll be able to hold your breath longer.

4. Recovery Breath: When you must breathe, take one big inhale and hold the breath for 10 to 15 seconds before exhaling. You can check the stopwatch to see your breath hold duration.

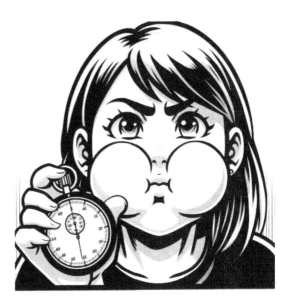

5. Repetition: Repeat steps 2 through 4 for another 2 rounds.

At the end of 3 total sequences, return to a normal breathing pattern and relax or meditate for a few minutes, soaking up any feelings of warmth, love, and power from within.

Wim Hof emphasizes the importance of mental resilience. By teaching your body to relax around the sensation of needing something immediately, such as air, you can extend this practice to other areas of life. This approach fosters patience, endurance, and the ability to remain calm in stressful situations. Embracing discomfort and delayed gratification has the potential to lead to great rewards, helping you achieve a more balanced and fulfilling life.

The Wim Hof Method is highly efficient and can be integrated into a busy daily routine, making it ideal for today's lifestyle. You are welcome to do additional rounds, but with only 93 breaths in 3 rounds taking less than 15 minutes to complete, you can put yourself in an incredible mindset for a fantastic day. The Wim Hof Method is known for its ability to boost energy levels, enhance focus, reduce stress, and improve the immune response. Combining this breathing technique with cold exposure (such as cold showers or ice baths) can further enhance its benefits.

Buteyko Method: Breathing for Optimal Oxygenation

The Buteyko Method, developed by Dr. Konstantin Buteyko, focuses on reducing over-breathing and improving oxygenation at the cellular level. This method is particularly beneficial for people with respiratory conditions such as asthma. The basic principles of the Buteyko Method include:

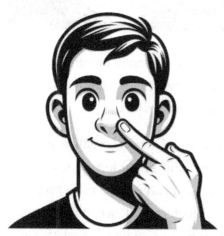

1. Nose Breathing: Breathe through your nose at all times, both day and night.

2. Breath Volume Reduction: Reduce the volume of each breath to normalize breathing patterns and increase carbon dioxide levels in the blood.

3. Build Up CO2 Tolerance: Practice specific breath-holding exercises such as the one described on the next page to improve your tolerance to carbon dioxide.

Buteyko Exercise: One common Buteyko exercise involves the following steps:

1. Position: Sit in a comfortable position and breathe normally through your nose.

2. Exhale: After a natural exhalation, pinch your nose and hold your breath.

3. Breath Hold: Hold your breath until you feel a strong urge to breathe, then release your nose and breathe normally through your nose again.

4. Repeat: Repeat several times, gradually increasing the breath-hold duration as your CO_2 tolerance improves.

The Buteyko Method aims to retrain the respiratory system, reduce symptoms of chronic overbreathing, and improve overall respiratory health.

Holotropic Breathwork: Unlocking Deep Inner Healing

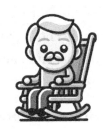

Holotropic Breathwork, developed by Dr. Stanislav Grof and Christina Grof, is a powerful technique designed to access deeper levels of the psyche and facilitate profound emotional and psychological healing. It is the granddaddy of Somatic Release and Transformational Breathwork and has similarities to Rebirthing Breathwork developed in the 1970s by Leonard Orr. This method involves rapid and deep breathing for 3 hours combined with evocative music to induce an altered state of consciousness. The term "holotropic" comes from the Greek words "holos" (whole) and "trepein" (to move toward), meaning "moving toward wholeness."

How to Practice Holotropic Breathwork

Holotropic Breathwork sessions are facilitated by trained practitioners in a controlled and safe environment. This is not an everyday event. Here's a basic outline of what you can expect during a session:

1. Preparation: Before starting, participants often engage in a brief meditation or grounding exercise to center themselves. The facilitator explains the process and sets the intention for the session.

2. Breathing Technique: Participants lie down in a comfortable position and begin to breathe rapidly and deeply. The breathing pattern is continuous and connected, with no pauses between the inhale and exhale.

3. Music: Evocative and rhythmic music is played to guide the journey. The music is carefully chosen to support the emotional and energetic flow of the session.

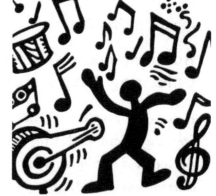

4. State of Consciousness: As the breathing continues, participants may enter an altered state of consciousness. This state can bring up vivid memories, emotions, and sensations, often leading to profound insights and healing experiences.

5. Integration: After the breathing session, participants spend time integrating their experiences. This may involve journaling, drawing, or discussing their journey with the facilitator and other participants.

Benefits of Holotropic Breathwork

Holotropic Breathwork is known for its potential to facilitate deep inner work and transformation. Some of the benefits include:

Emotional Release: This technique can help release pent-up emotions and unresolved trauma, allowing for deep emotional healing.

Self-Discovery: Participants often gain insights into their subconscious mind, uncovering hidden aspects of themselves and their life experiences.

Stress Reduction: The process can lead to a profound sense of relaxation and stress relief, promoting overall well-being.

Spiritual Connection: Many participants report experiencing a sense of connection to a higher power or a greater sense of purpose and meaning in life.

Enhanced Creativity: The altered state of consciousness can unlock creative potential and new ways of thinking.

Important Considerations

Holotropic Breathwork is a powerful practice that should be approached with care and respect. It is recommended to work with a trained facilitator who can provide a safe and supportive environment. This technique may not be suitable for everyone, particularly those with certain medical conditions such as cardiovascular issues, severe mental illness, or epilepsy. Always consult with a healthcare professional before starting any new Breathwork practice.

Holotropic Breathwork offers a unique and transformative approach to exploring the depths of the psyche and promoting holistic healing. By engaging in this practice, we can uncover profound insights, release emotional blockages, and move toward greater wholeness and well-being.

The Science of Smiling: How a Grin Boosts Happiness

Smiling has a profound impact on our well-being, primarily by triggering the release of several key "feel-good" hormones. When we smile—whether we are feeling happy or not—our brain releases dopamine, serotonin, and endorphins. These chemicals play a significant role in enhancing our mood, reducing stress, and even alleviating pain.

Dopamine is often referred to as the "reward hormone" because it creates feelings of pleasure and satisfaction. Serotonin works as a natural mood lifter, similar to the way many antidepressants function, but without any negative side effects. Endorphins act as natural painkillers, providing an analgesic effect that can reduce physical discomfort—this gives a whole new meaning to "Grin and bear it."

Moreover, the benefits of smiling aren't limited to personal well-being. Smiling can improve your social interactions, making you appear more approachable and trustworthy, which helps in forming and strengthening social bonds. The contagious nature of smiling means that when you smile, others are likely to smile back, creating a positive feedback loop of happiness and connection.

Incorporating more smiles into your daily life can also lead to improved physical health. Smiling and laughing can lower your heart rate and blood pressure, contributing to a relaxed state that counters the effects of stress. Over time, this can lead to better overall health and longevity.

Forcing a smile can even trick your brain into feeling happier, a concept often summarized by the phrase "fake it till you make it." This means that even if you don't feel happy, consciously smiling can help improve your mood and lead to genuine feelings of happiness over time.

Smiling Leads to Laughter: The Most Fun Breathwork of All

Laughter is often described as the best medicine, and for good reason. It offers a multitude of health advantages, both physical and psychological, and can be an enjoyable form of Breathwork. Engaging in laughter exercises can produce positive health benefits, even if the laughter isn't in response to something humorous. The goal is to promote health and well-being through voluntary laughter. Some health Benefits of laughter include:

Reduces Stress and Enhances Mood: Laughter triggers the release of endorphins, the body's natural feel-good chemicals, promoting an overall sense of well-being and temporarily relieving pain. It also decreases the levels of stress hormones like cortisol and adrenaline, helping us feel more relaxed and less stressed.

Boosts the Immune System: Laughter increases the production of antibodies and activates immune cells, thereby improving our resistance to disease. A stronger immune system means better overall health and a reduced risk of illness.

Improves Cardiovascular Health: Laughing enhances blood flow, which can help protect us against heart attacks and other cardiovascular problems. It improves the function of blood vessels and increases blood flow, which can help prevent heart disease.

Provides a Natural Workout: Laughter exercises the diaphragm, contracts the abs, and even works out the shoulders, leaving muscles more relaxed afterward. It also provides a good cardio workout, increasing our heart rate and burning calories.

Relieves Pain: Through the release of endorphins, laughter can provide natural pain relief. It also distracts from pain and can help people tolerate discomfort better.

Laughter Exercises:

Laughter exercises involve various activities designed to stimulate laughter. These might include deep breathing exercises followed by forced laughter, playful behaviors, and laughter yoga, 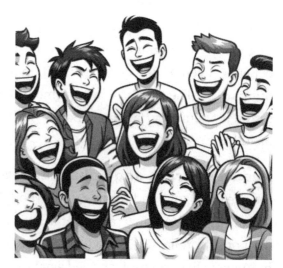 which combines laughter exercises with yoga breathing techniques. Here are a few examples you can do on your own with more group laughter exercises to come:

Ho-Ha-Hum Exercise: Start by saying "Ho" deep in the belly, then move up to the chest to say "Ha," followed by "Hum" up in the nose in a rhythmic pattern and then keep going. Be sure to smile.

Laughing Alone: Stand in front of a mirror and practice laughing at yourself. This can often lead to genuine laughter.

Laughter Meditation: Sit comfortably, take a few deep breaths, and then start to laugh. Allow the laughter to come naturally and let it flow for several minutes.

Laughter Yoga America

Sebastien Gendry is the C.E.O. of the American School of Laughter Yoga and a leading Laughter Yoga expert in the world. I find his Laughter Yoga Exercises easy and fun to do. Try them!

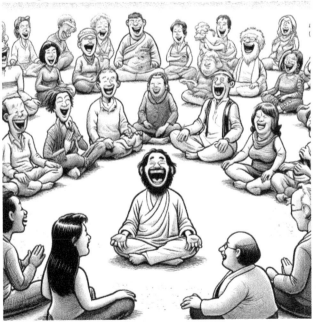

20 Laughter Yoga Exercises: By Sebastien Gendry

Here are 20 laughter yoga exercises categorized into five groups to help you begin your laughter journey. Some of these exercises can be practiced alone but they are designed to be practiced with others, fostering social connection and enhancing the overall experience. Remember, choosing to laugh when you want is a sign of maturity, not silliness. Give these exercises at least 10 minutes, and you'll notice a shift in your mood state.

5 Classic Laughter Yoga Exercises

1. Cell Phone Laughter: Hold an imaginary cell phone to your ear and laugh.

2. Gradient Laughter: Fake a smile, giggle, then laugh slowly and gradually increase in tempo and volume.

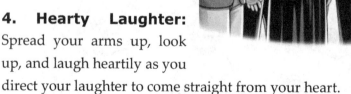

3. Greeting Laughter: Greet everybody the way you normally greet (e.g., shake hands) and replace words with laughter.

4. Hearty Laughter: Spread your arms up, look up, and laugh heartily as you direct your laughter to come straight from your heart.

5. Awkward Situation Laughter: Think of a socially awkward situation (e.g., untied shoelaces, shaving cream behind your ears) and laugh at it.

5 Laughter Yoga Exercises to Release Stress:

1. Argument Laughter: Voice your discontent in laughter sounds only, or in pig-latin. You can be as passionate as you'd like and point fingers if you want, just don't hit (or even threaten to hit) anything or anybody.

2. Credit Card Bill Laughter: Open an imaginary credit card bill (or any other letter that represents bad news to you) and burst out laughing the second you look at what's inside.

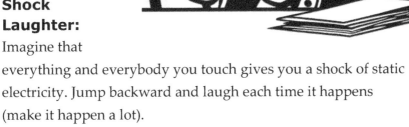

3. Electric Shock Laughter: Imagine that everything and everybody you touch gives you a shock of static electricity. Jump backward and laugh each time it happens (make it happen a lot).

4. I Don't Know Why I Am Laughing: Laugh (fake is perfectly fine) and shrug your shoulders and make a big smile as you look at yourself in a mirror or anybody else who might be there and try to convey the message with your eyes and body language "I absolutely don't know why I am laughing".

5. No Money Laughter: Laugh as you turn your pockets inside out looking for money that isn't there.

5 Laughter Yoga Exercises Acting As Children:

1. Baby Laughter: One person must demonstrate how a baby laughs (take turns!). Everybody else must then do the same thing.

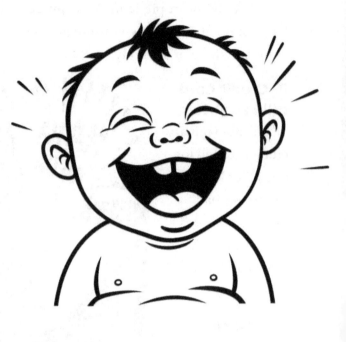

2. Favorite Animal Laughter: Laugh and behave the way your favorite animal or pet would behave if it was very happy to see you.

3. Chicken Laughter: Imagine you are a chicken. First, lay 3 eggs in 3 laughs, then laugh with lots of excitement in your voice as you go tell the world about it.

4. Jumping Frog: Squat down, hands on the floor between your knees. Jump once saying "ha", then a second time saying "ha ha", a third time saying "ha ha ha", then jump in fast succession laughing a lot.

5. Laughter Vowels: Let's learn the laughter vowels! Start with "A" as in "hat": Aaaaa ha ha ha ha ha. Next is "E" as in "hen": Eeeee he he he he he. Next is "I" as in "hiccup": Iiiii hi hi hi hi hi. Next is "O" as in "Otto": Ooooo ho ho ho ho ho. Last is "U" as in "soup": Uuuuu hu hu hu hu hu.

5 Laughter Yoga Exercises for Seniors:

1. Back Pain Laughter: Lean forward and put your hand on your lower back, then laugh as if you could not stand back up.

2. Conductor Laughter: Imagine you are a conductor. Direct an imaginary orchestra with enthusiastic arm movements as you sing any song of your choice in laughter sounds only (e.g., ho ho ho or ha ha ha).

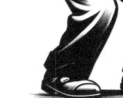

3.   Ear-Wiggle Laughter: Slowly slide your left hand upward along the left side of your head, slowly going over your head as you say an extended "aeeee" sound, then laugh as you wiggle your right ear with your left fingers. Do the same on the other side. Repeat a few times.

4. Laughter Pill: Take some imaginary laughter pills! Each pill has a unique effect and makes you laugh and jerk in a peculiar way for just a few seconds. Try another one as soon as the effects wear off.

5. Vowel Movement Laughter: Have you had your vowel movement today? Laugh in the tonality of the following sounds: Eee Eee Eee Eee! Aye aye aye aye! Ah ah ah ah! Ho ho ho ho! Ooo ooo ooo ooo! Uh uh uh uh!

Many of these exercises can be done alone or in groups, making it easy to incorporate laughter into your daily routine. The contagious nature of laughter means that even simulated laughter can quickly become real, creating a joyful and healthy environment for everyone involved. So, let the giggles begin and try incorporating laughter exercises into daily interactions with family members, coworkers, and friends. It's fun, effective, and a wonderful way to bond with others.

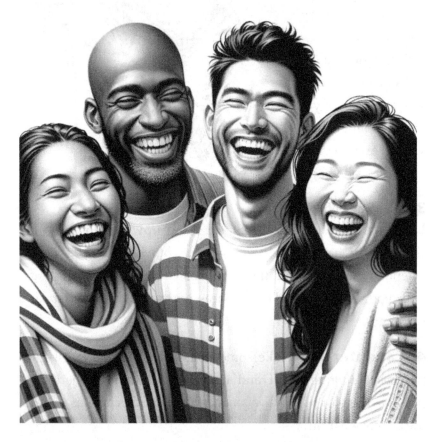

Resources for Further Exploration

This chapter provides a glimpse into the diverse world of Breathwork techniques but only scratches the surface. Each of these techniques could have an entire book written about it, and many of them do. To dive deeper into any of these methods and research additional modalities, refer to the resources provided at the end of this book and on the website TheBreathMD.com. Exploring these resources will allow us to expand our Breathwork practice and discover even more ways to harness the power of our breath for long-term stress relief and overall well-being.

8
INTEGRATING BREATH INTO DAILY LIFE

"The time to relax is when you don't have time for it."
- Sydney J. Harris

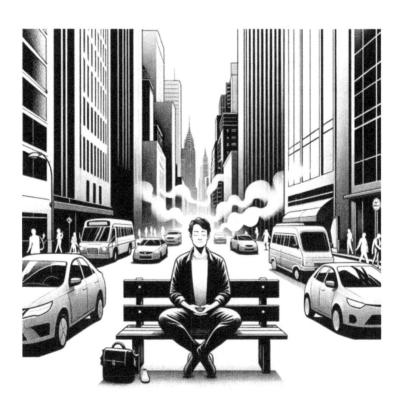

Creating a Breath-Centered Lifestyle

Integrating breath into our daily lives can have profound effects on our overall well-being. It's not just about practicing Breathwork techniques during designated meditation sessions— it's about bringing awareness to our breath in every moment and using it as a tool to navigate life's ups and downs. Here are some ways to create a breath-centered lifestyle:

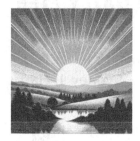

Start Your Day with Breathwork: Begin each morning with a few minutes of deep breathing or mindful breathing. This can help set a positive tone for the day ahead and provide a sense of calm and centeredness.

Practice Mindfulness Throughout the Day: Bring awareness to your breath as you go about your daily activities. Notice the sensation of the air entering and leaving your body, the rise and fall of your chest or abdomen, and any other sensations associated with breathing. This can help anchor you in the present moment and reduce stress and anxiety.

Use Breath as a Tool for Stress Management: Whenever you feel stressed or overwhelmed, take a few moments to focus on your breath. Try taking slow, deep breaths or using a specific Breathwork technique like diaphragmatic breathing or alternate nostril breathing. This can help activate the body's relaxation response and calm your mind and body.

Incorporate Breathwork into Everyday Tasks: Look for opportunities to incorporate Breathwork into your daily routine. For example, you can practice deep breathing while waiting in line at the grocery store or take a few mindful breaths before responding to an email or phone call. By integrating Breathwork into everyday tasks, you can make it a natural and effortless part of your life.

Use Breath as a Tool for Self-Care: Make time for regular Breathwork practice as part of your self-care routine. Whether it's through guided meditation, yoga, or simply taking a few moments to focus on your breath, prioritize self-care practices that nourish your mind, body, and spirit.

By creating a breath-centered lifestyle, you can cultivate greater awareness, resilience, and well-being in your daily life. Remember that it's not about perfection—it's about finding moments throughout the day to pause, breathe, and reconnect with yourself.

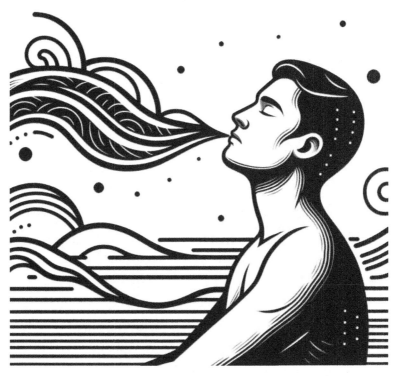

The Importance of Grounding

In our stressed out modern society, we can go weeks to months without ever touching our feet to the Earth. This never happened when we lived in tribes. It turns out, our physical bodies made of cells with electrical charges do not work as well without resetting by contacting the ground. Grounding, also known as earthing, refers to the practice of making direct physical contact with the Earth, such as walking barefoot on natural surfaces like grass, sand, or soil. It can be combined with Breathwork and movement for additional benefits.

Direct skin contact is best for grounding although there is evidence emerging that you can ground through any material that conducts such as through leather moccasins or on a blanket on the ground (often important in Tennessee due to chiggers, hookworms, and other biting insects in the grass) or even through concrete (as long as you are not wearing rubber soled shoes which do not conduct).

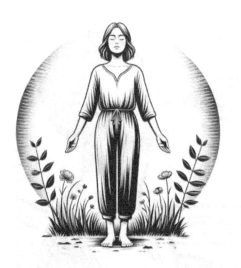

This practice can act like a reset of our cells combating feelings of stress and anxiety. Most of the research studies tested twenty to thirty minutes of ground contact, but even a few minutes may be beneficial.

Grounding intentionally connects you with the Earth's electromagnetic energy, offering numerous health benefits.

Scientific Facts and Studies on Grounding

There is science to back up the idea that our physical bodies perform better after contacting the ground. Our bodies accumulate positive charges due to various sources, such as electronic devices, synthetic materials, and electromagnetic fields (EMFs). The Earth has a negative charge due to its abundance of free electrons. When we come into direct contact with the Earth, we allow these electrons to flow into our bodies, helping to balance our internal electrical state. When we are not grounded, our bodies can carry a higher electrical potential relative to the Earth which can lead to the build up of static electricity and other electrical imbalances. Free radicals, which are positively charged molecules, are associated with inflammation and oxidative stress in the body. The influx of free electrons from the Earth can neutralize these free radicals, reducing oxidative stress and inflammation resulting in better health. Here are some of the benefits of grounding:

Reduction of Inflammation and Pain: A study published in the *Journal of Inflammation Research* found that grounding reduces inflammation and pain. The study showed that grounding influences the immune system by reducing various markers of inflammation, including white blood cell count and cytokine production. By reducing inflammation and oxidative stress, grounding supports the immune system, making it more effective in fighting off infections and diseases. Grounding has been shown to significantly reduce the levels of inflammatory markers by up to 20% in just a few hours of practice. Grounding can be an effective natural method for managing chronic pain, particularly in conditions like arthritis and muscle soreness.

Improved Sleep: Research published in the *Journal of Alternative and Complementary Medicine* demonstrated that grounding during sleep can improve sleep quality. Participants who slept on grounded mattress pads experienced better sleep, reduced pain, and increased feelings of well-being. Grounding promotes deeper and more restful sleep, which is crucial for overall health and recovery. Over 85% of participants in grounding studies reported better sleep quality and fewer sleep disturbances.

Stress Reduction and Mood Enhancement: Grounding has been shown to reduce stress and improve mood. A pilot study published in *Psychological Reports* (2011) found that grounding significantly reduced stress levels and enhanced mood by balancing cortisol levels, a key hormone involved in the stress response. By balancing cortisol levels and promoting relaxation, grounding helps in managing stress and enhancing emotional well-being. Studies have found that grounding can reduce cortisol levels by up to 30%, leading to a more balanced stress response .

Improved Blood Flow: A study published in *The Journal of Alternative and Complementary Medicine* found that grounding improves blood flow and circulation. The study noted that grounding increases the surface charge of red blood cells, reducing blood viscosity and improving overall cardiovascular health. Improved blood flow and reduced blood viscosity contribute to better cardiovascular health by lowering the risk of heart-related conditions. Grounding can increase blood flow and reduce blood viscosity by approximately 30%, improving cardiovascular function. Better blood flow is also important for wound healing.

Reduction of Electromagnetic Fields (EMFs)

Impact: Grounding has been suggested to mitigate the adverse effects of exposure to electromagnetic fields (EMFs). A study published in the *Journal of Environmental and Public Health* showed that grounding helps reduce the impact of EMFs on the body by neutralizing positive electrons and promoting a healthier electrical state in the body.

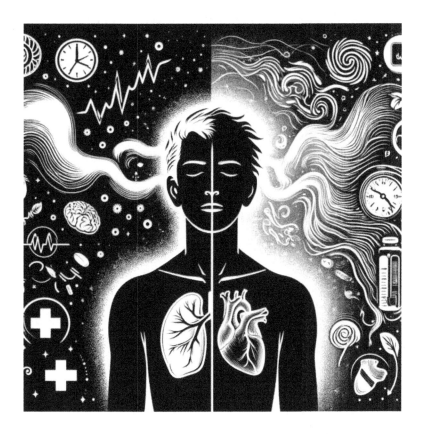

How Grounding Works and Its Best Practices

Grounding is like rebooting your computer. Just as rebooting clears out the glitches and resets the system, grounding helps to reset your body's electrical state, promoting optimal health and well-being. It can be done standing up or sitting down.

The best way to ground is to have your bare feet on the Earth. Natural surfaces like grass, sand, or soil are ideal because they are highly conductive. However, you can still ground yourself by standing on other conductive materials like concrete, provided you are not wearing rubber-soled shoes, which do not conduct electricity. Saltwater is particularly conductive, so standing barefoot in saltwater can enhance the grounding effect.

Bare feet on the ground is better than bare feet on concrete, but this is akin to eating organic versus non-organic vegetables: eating organic is preferable, but consuming non-organic is still beneficial compared to not eating vegetables at all. While there is less scientific evidence supporting grounding on indoor concrete, being outdoors is generally better because our brains are wired for nature, including sunshine, birds singing, plants, and trees.

Visualization Techniques for Grounding

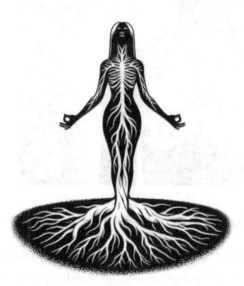

Grounding can also be enhanced through visualization techniques. These are optional as simply standing on the ground offers health benefits but in the face of chronic stress and anxiety, reinforcing being connected to something bigger than oneself can put worries in perspective. Try it out and see what works best for you.

One technique is to imagine a tree's roots growing from the base of your spine through your legs going deep into the Earth— going down, down, down, reaching the Earth's center. Feel your connection with the center of the Earth seeing its red core energy coming up to nourish your body.

Another visualization is to imagine a thick rope with a huge hook on the end going down from the base of your spine into the ground, going down, down, down until it reaches the center of the Earth and then the hook hooks in place. Imagine you actually feel the hook lock in place with a little tug as you are completely connected to the Earth.

Movements Tied to the Exhale and Inhale

Once visualizing a tie between yourself and the center of the Earth, incorporating the following movements can be helpful when grounding as it increases your connection with nature while allowing your body to move and stretch. Inhale imagining bringing the Earth's energy up into your body as your hands rise to release to the sky and on the exhale bring the sky's energy down into your body and back to the Earth. Do this for at least 10 rounds to feel the amazing calming effects of moving with the breath. Here's how the sequence flows:

1. Stand Tall: With feet together, arms at your sides, and weight evenly distributed on your feet.

2. Exhale and Hinge at Your Hips: Fold forward, bringing your hands toward the ground, as your legs stretch.

3. Visualize: While folded forward, visualize scooping up energy from the Earth with your hands bringing the energy up the front side of your body.

4. Inhale: As you rise up, raising your arms overhead, reaching up and feeling the energy rise with you.

5. Exhale: Bring your straightened arms in a circle back down to your sides while you visualize bringing white light down through your body.

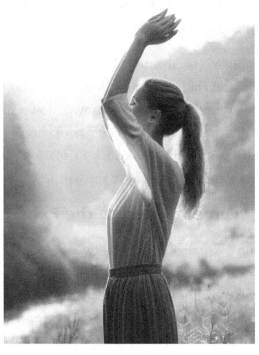

6. Repeat: Then fold at the waist and repeat from step 2.

Inhaling and exhaling while moving in this flowing movement results in getting the blood pumping, stretching the body, and calming the mind while enjoying the benefits of grounding. By integrating grounding into daily life, you can harness the Earth's natural energy to reboot and rejuvenate your body and mind.

Breathwork for Specific Situations: Work, Relationships, and Challenging Circumstances

Breathwork can be a valuable tool for navigating specific situations in our lives, from the workplace to our relationships to challenging circumstances. By using Breathwork techniques tailored to the situation at hand, we can manage stress, improve communication, and cultivate greater resilience. Our breath can act as a remote control to calm ourselves in the moment, allowing us to increase the pause between events and our responses. The more we can increase this pause, the more we are able to consciously choose our actions. Any of the Breathwork techniques we have already discussed in this book can be helpful in multiple different areas of life. One technique is not necessarily better than another. Experiment and discover what is most beneficial for you. Here are some ideas of how to use Breathwork in specific situations:

Work

Many of us experience stress and pressure in our work lives, whether it's meeting deadlines, dealing with difficult coworkers, or navigating organizational changes. Breathwork can help us stay calm and focused in the face of work-related stress while improving overall productivity. Here are several suggestions for using Breathwork when stressed at work:

1. Dealing with a Difficult Coworker:

- Example: If a coworker's behavior is consistently aggravating or disrespectful, it can be hard to maintain your composure.

- Breathwork Technique: Use 4-4-6 breathing to calm your nervous system and manage your emotional responses. Begin by inhaling deeply for four seconds, holding the breath for four seconds, and then exhaling slowly for six seconds. This technique helps to regulate your stress response and maintain a sense of control.

You can practice 4-4-6 breathing subtly at your desk, in the restroom, or even in the moment without being detected. By focusing on your breath, you can create a buffer between your

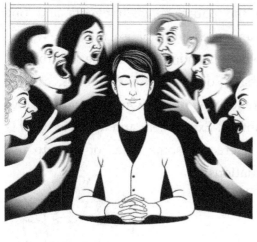

emotional reactions and the coworker's triggering behavior.

Regularly using this Breathwork technique allows you to stay composed and centered, even in challenging interactions. It helps you respond to

aggravating or disrespectful behavior with calmness and clarity, maintaining your professionalism and emotional balance.

2. Responding to an Overbearing Supervisor:

- Example: When a supervisor is micromanaging or giving constant negative feedback, it can create a lot of stress.

- Breathwork Technique: Practice coherent breathing to stay balanced. Breathe in for five seconds and then breathe out for five seconds while bringing focus to your heart and generating gratitude—consider being grateful you have a job that allows you to pay the bills. This technique helps you maintain a calm and composed state, even when facing stressful situations. You can practice this during a meeting or while listening to triggering feedback.

Additionally, try to mentally visualize your supervisor in a humorous way, such as imagining them in their underwear or farting in public. Remember that this person puts their pants on one leg at a time just like everyone else. This mental trick can help you humanize them and reduce the intensity of their overbearing behavior.

By combining coherent breathing with a lighthearted perspective, you can manage your stress levels, respond more effectively, and maintain your emotional equilibrium in the face of micromanagement and negative feedback.

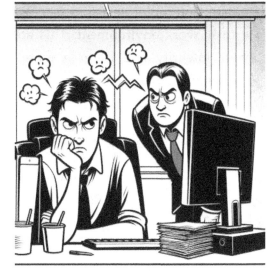

3. Surviving a Negative Work Environment:

- Example: A toxic work culture with gossip, blame, and negativity can be draining.

- Breathwork Technique: Use box breathing to reset your stress response and maintain your composure. Inhale for four seconds, hold for four seconds, exhale for four seconds, and hold for another four seconds. Take short breaks throughout the day to practice this technique, helping you stay centered amidst the negativity.

Additionally, avoid participating in gossip. While it may seem like joining in negative talk about the boss or colleagues scores you points with the group, it actually signals to others that you talk behind people's backs. This behavior undermines your trustworthiness, whether or not others consciously realize it. Limiting your exposure to such negativity is crucial, as it will only bring you down.

By consistently practicing box breathing and steering clear of gossip, you can protect your mental and emotional well-being in a toxic work environment. This approach helps you maintain your integrity and foster a more positive mindset, even in challenging circumstances.

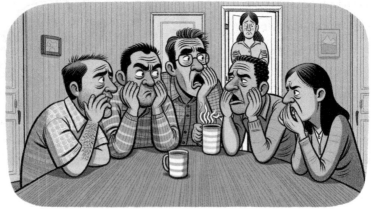

4. Enduring Conflict with a Team Member:

- Example: If you have ongoing conflicts with a team member, it can affect your productivity and mental health.

- Breathwork Technique: Try mindful breathing by focusing on the natural rhythm of your breath. This can help you remain calm and respond thoughtfully rather than reacting emotionally. Inhale deeply and exhale slowly, paying close attention to the flow of your breath. This practice helps center your mind and reduce stress.

Additionally, make an effort to truly listen and see the situation from your team member's point of view. Ask yourself: What do they truly want? What is their motivation? Understanding their perspective can enable you to develop a win-win solution. It takes two to fight, but instead of fighting, strive for a greater good by seeking common ground.

By combining mindful breathing with empathetic listening, you can manage conflicts more effectively. This approach helps you stay composed and fosters a collaborative environment where both parties can work towards mutually beneficial outcomes.

5. Meeting Unreasonable Deadlines:

- Example: When facing unrealistic deadlines and the pressure feels overwhelming.

- Breathwork Technique: Practice deep diaphragmatic breathing to reduce anxiety and stay focused on your tasks. Inhale deeply into your diaphragm, hold for a moment, and exhale slowly. This technique helps calm your mind and body, allowing you to approach your work with a clear head.

Additionally, visualize the work already done. Imagine what it feels like to have completed the task, how good it feels to have it behind you. Picture yourself having more than enough time to not only meet the deadline but to do so with ease and exceed expectations. This positive visualization can help propel you towards your goal, enhancing your motivation and efficiency.

By combining deep diaphragmatic breathing with positive visualization, you can manage the stress of unreasonable deadlines more effectively. This approach helps you stay calm, focused, and driven, ensuring that you can tackle your tasks with confidence and achieve outstanding results.

Relationships

Breathwork can also be helpful in improving our relationships with others. By practicing mindful breathing, we can become more present and attentive in our interactions with loved ones, fostering deeper connections and communication. Here are several suggestions for using Breathwork when dealing with triggering situations in relationships:

1. Before a Difficult Conversation with a Partner:

- Example: When discussing a sensitive topic with your partner, emotions can run high, leading to arguments or misunderstandings. How you start the conversation can make all the difference.

- Breathwork Technique: Start with grounding as described earlier in this chapter to anchor yourself in the present moment. Then, practice coherent breathing by inhaling for five seconds and exhaling for five seconds. Focus on breathing into your

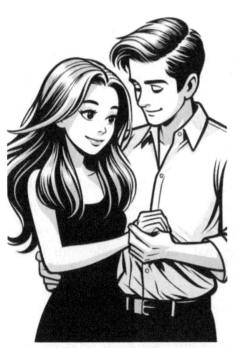

heart, generating feelings of gratitude and appreciation. Reflect on all the reasons you are with your partner, acknowledging the good and the vulnerability of this person.

Visualize the positive aspects of your relationship and the love you share. This mental shift can transform the emotional landscape of your conversation, helping you approach the discussion with empathy and understanding. By setting this compassionate tone before the conversation begins, you create a more open and respectful environment, which can significantly alter how the discussion unfolds.

This Breathwork technique not only calms your mind but also fosters a deeper connection with your partner, making it easier to navigate sensitive topics with grace and mutual respect.

2. Conflict with a Family Member:

- Example: Family gatherings can sometimes bring up old conflicts and unresolved issues, making it hard to stay calm.

- Breathwork Technique: Practice 4-4-6 breathing during moments of tension: inhale for four seconds, hold for four seconds, and exhale for six seconds. This technique helps you stay grounded and calm amidst the chaos, allowing you to be the eye of the storm.

Remember the power of the pause before speaking. Often, we feel pressure to fill the silence, and what we say may not be well thought out, potentially adding fuel to the fire. Instead, take a moment to pause and breathe, allowing your words to come from a higher place—or choose to say nothing at all.

Sometimes, choosing peace over being right is a better path in the long run. This Breathwork technique enables you to approach conflicts with a calm and clear mind, reducing the likelihood of escalation and fostering a more harmonious environment.

3. Parenting Stress:

- Example: Managing tantrums or behavioral issues with children can be very stressful and triggering.

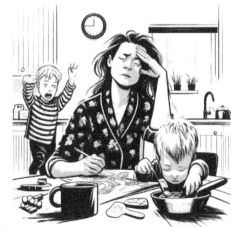

- Breathwork Technique: Try incorporating laughter into these challenging moments. Use any of the laughter exercises discussed earlier to bring lightness to the situation. Remember, kids are just kids, and responding to their tantrums with your own tantrum will not improve the situation. Instead, laugh.

When you choose to laugh, it can shift the energy in the room, surprising your children and potentially stopping their crying. They might even start laughing with you. This unexpected response can defuse the tension and create a more positive atmosphere, making it easier to handle the stress of parenting with a sense of humor and perspective.

4. Tension with Friends:

- Example: Misunderstandings or disagreements with friends can create tension and stress in your relationship.

- Breathwork Technique: Before meeting up with your friends, take a moment to practice mindful breathing by focusing on the natural rhythm of your breath. Calm your body and reflect on how you feel after spending time with them. Do they uplift you or bring you down? This can be a challenging question because the answer might reveal that you have outgrown some of your old friends, signaling it's time to make new connections.

As you evolve, old friends may no longer align with who you are becoming, and that's okay—no judgment. They have the right to remain where they are, but you have the power to move forward. Choose to spend your time with people who respect and appreciate your growth. By practicing mindful breathing and reflecting on your friendships, you can navigate tensions with clarity and make choices that support your well-being and personal development.

5. Dealing with a Critical In-Law:

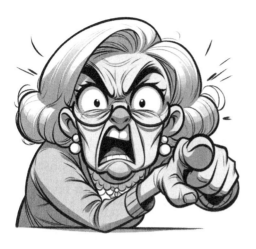

- Example: Interactions with a critical or judgmental in-law can be emotionally draining and triggering.

- Breathwork Technique: Before meeting with your in-law, find a quiet space and close your eyes. Visualize your in-law as a child who has experienced trauma or hardship, contributing to a critical nature. Understand that their behavior stems from their own pain and is not a reflection of you. This visualization helps cultivate compassion and perspective, making it easier to handle their criticism without internalizing it.

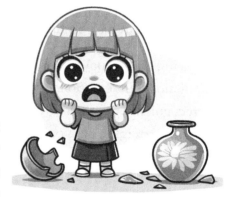

Next, practice box breathing to calm your mind and body. Inhale deeply through your nose for a count of four. Hold your breath for another count of four. Exhale slowly through your mouth for a count of four. Hold your breath again for a count of four. Repeat this cycle until you feel calm. Box breathing helps regulate your nervous system, preparing you to face the interaction with a sense of calm and control.

During the interaction, if you start to feel overwhelmed, discreetly practice box breathing. This can help you stay calm

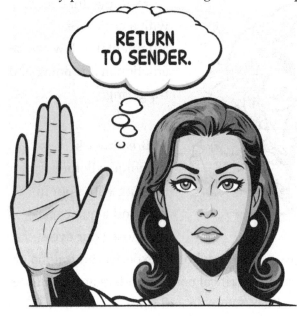

and composed even in the face of criticism. When your in-law speaks harshly or critically, listen to your heart and remind yourself that these words do not define you. Mentally say to yourself,

"Return to Sender," acknowledging that the negative energy and words are not yours to accept and sending them back to the person from whom they originated.

By practicing this visualization and Breathwork technique, you can maintain your emotional balance and protect your inner peace, recognizing that their words and behavior are reflections of their own struggles, not your worth.

Challenging Circumstances

When faced with challenging circumstances or adversity, Breathwork can provide a sense of stability and resilience. By connecting with our breath, we can anchor ourselves in the present moment and tap into our inner resources for strength and courage. Here are several suggestions for using Breathwork when dealing with challenging circumstances:

1. Facing a Major Life Change:

- Example: Moving to a new city, starting a new job, or ending a significant relationship can be overwhelming and stressful.

- Breathwork Technique: Use visualization and Breathwork to navigate this challenging time. Begin by taking a few moments to visualize the new situation working out great and exactly how you want it to. Take time to think about what you truly desire and what the best possible outcome would be.

Once you have a clear vision, practice coherent breathing to balance your nervous system. Inhale deeply for five seconds, and then exhale for five seconds breathing from your heart. Continue this cycle, focusing on maintaining a steady rhythm. This practice helps to calm your mind and body, enabling you to face the new life change with a sense of balance and tranquility.

By combining visualization with coherent breathing, you can create a mental and physical state that supports your ability to overcome obstacles and navigate difficult situations with grace and ease. This approach not only reduces stress but also empowers you to approach major life changes with confidence and a positive mindset.

2. Dealing with Health Issues:

- Example: Coping with a serious illness or recovering from an injury can be physically and emotionally draining.

- Breathwork Technique: Use deep diaphragmatic breathing combined with body awareness to support your healing process. Begin by inhaling deeply into your diaphragm, allowing your belly to expand fully. Hold the breath for a moment, and then exhale slowly, letting all the tension release from your body.

While practicing this breathing technique, engage in a mental body scan. Start from the top of your head and move down to your toes, paying attention to any areas of tension, discomfort, or pain. Listen to your body and acknowledge what it is telling you. Recognize your body as an integral part of you with its own needs and signals.

As you continue to breathe deeply, generate a sense of gratitude for how your body serves you, despite its current challenges. Appreciate the resilience and strength it shows in the face of illness or injury. Cultivate gratitude for being alive and having the opportunity to heal and recover.

This practice not only calms your mind and nervous system but also fosters a compassionate and appreciative relationship with your body, enhancing your overall sense of well-being during difficult times.

3. Financial Stress:

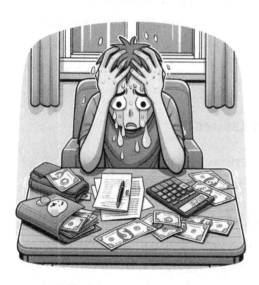

- Example: Struggling with financial difficulties, such as debt or job loss, can create a significant amount of stress and worry.

- Breathwork Technique: Use coherent breathing to find balance and calm amidst financial stress. Begin by breathing in for a count of five seconds and then exhaling for a count of five seconds. After a few cycles, reverse the count: inhale for one second, then two, three, four, and finally five. Then, exhale for five seconds, four, three, two, and finally one. Continue this pattern, getting into a rhythm and a flow state.

As you find your rhythm and balance, shift your focus to gratitude. Reflect on all the things you currently have in your life that you are thankful for. Bask in this feeling of gratitude, allowing it to fill your mind and heart. As your mind clears and your body relaxes, you may find that ideas and inspirations begin to emerge.

Sometimes, solutions to your financial challenges that you hadn't considered before can appear when you are in this balanced state. By combining coherent breathing with gratitude, you create a mental space conducive to innovative thinking and problem-solving, helping you navigate financial stress with a clearer mind and a more positive outlook.

4. Handling Grief and Loss:

- Example: The loss of a loved one or a significant life change can bring about intense feelings of grief and sadness.

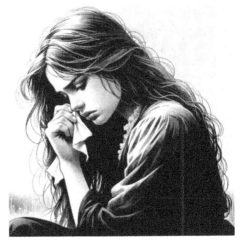

- Breathwork Technique: Somatic Release Breathwork and Transformational Breathwork can lead to major breakthroughs when dealing with grief and loss. These types of Breathwork help release deeply held emotions and allow you to reach a new perspective, which can be particularly beneficial when it's hard to see any positive side or happiness in the future.

Somatic Release and Transformational Breathwork will allow any trapped, unprocessed emotions to surface and release. Let any emotions that arise be expressed without judgment. This process helps to clear emotional blockages and can be a powerful way to process grief.

As you engage in these Breathwork practices, you may experience a release of emotions that have been weighing you down. This can create space for new perspectives and insights, helping you to process your grief to find a sense of peace. Over time, you may find that Breathwork helps you move through your grief, opening the door to healing and a renewed sense of hope for the future.

5. Managing High-Stress Situations:

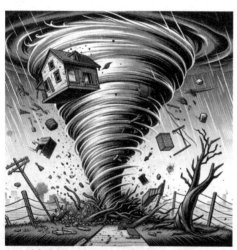

- Example: Experiencing a high-stress event such as a natural disaster, an accident, or a major conflict can be extremely challenging.

- Breathwork Technique: In high-stress situations, grounding yourself and using mindful breathing can help you stay present and calm immediately after the event. Begin with grounding exercises to anchor yourself in the present moment.

Feel your feet firmly planted on the ground, and take a few moments to connect with the physical sensations of your body.

Next, practice mindful breathing by focusing on the natural rhythm of your breath. Inhale deeply through your nose, filling your lungs completely, and then exhale slowly through your mouth. Pay close attention to the sensation of the breath entering and leaving your body. This focused breathing helps calm your mind and body, allowing you to remain composed and make clear decisions during and immediately after a crisis.

As you continue to breathe mindfully, remind yourself to stay present. Acknowledge any thoughts or emotions that arise, but let them pass without judgment. Return your focus to your breath, using it as a steady anchor in the midst of chaos.

Combining grounding with mindful breathing creates a powerful tool for managing high-stress situations. This approach helps you maintain clarity and composure, enabling you to respond effectively and thoughtfully to any challenges you face.

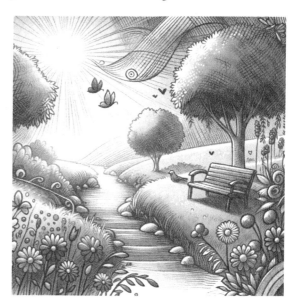

Other things to consider is that combining visualization with Breathwork to enhance its calming effects. Visualize a serene scene—go to your Happy Place—while practicing deep, slow breaths. In a stressful

217

situation, close your eyes and visualize a peaceful place while practicing coherent breathing. This can help you remain calm and centered, enabling you to handle the challenge with greater ease.

By incorporating these Breathwork techniques into our responses to challenging circumstances, we can better manage our emotional and physical reactions, leading to greater resilience and a more balanced approach to life's difficulties. We can enhance our ability to cope with stress, communicate effectively, and navigate life's challenges with greater ease and resilience.

Cultivating Resilience through Breath Awareness

Resilience is the ability to bounce back from adversity and overcome challenges with strength and flexibility. While some people may naturally possess more resilience than others, it's also a skill that can be cultivated and strengthened over time. Breath awareness is one

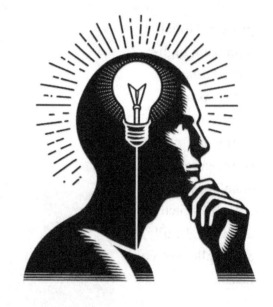

powerful tool for building resilience, as it helps us stay mentally grounded, centered, and calm in the face of adversity. Here's how to cultivate resilience through breath awareness:

Practice Mindfulness: Mindfulness is the practice of bringing focused attention to the present moment without judgment. By cultivating mindfulness through practices like mindful breathing, we can become more aware of our thoughts, feelings, and sensations, allowing us to respond to challenges with greater clarity and composure.

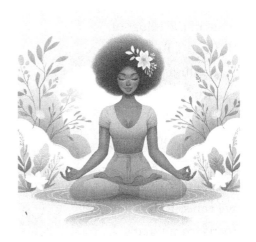

Develop Self-Awareness: Self-awareness is the ability to recognize and understand our own thoughts, feelings, and behaviors. By developing self-awareness through practices like Breathwork, we can identify our triggers and patterns of stress and develop healthier coping strategies.

Foster Self-Compassion: Self-compassion is the practice of treating ourselves with kindness, understanding, and acceptance, especially in times of difficulty or failure. By cultivating self-compassion through practices like loving-kindness meditation and self-soothing Breathwork techniques, we can build resilience and bounce back from setbacks with greater ease and grace.

Build a Support Network: Building a strong support network of friends, family, and community can also help bolster resilience. By connecting with others and sharing our experiences, we can gain perspective, encouragement, and practical support to help us navigate life's challenges.

Practice Gratitude: Gratitude is the practice of acknowledging and appreciating the good things in our lives, even in the midst of difficulty. By cultivating gratitude through practices like gratitude journaling and gratitude breathing exercises, we can shift our focus from what's lacking to what's present, fostering a sense of resilience and well-being.

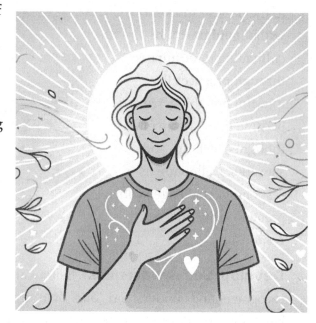

By cultivating resilience through breath awareness, we can build the inner strength and resources needed to navigate life's challenges with courage, grace, and resilience. Remember that resilience is a skill that can be developed and strengthened over time, and breath awareness is a powerful tool for building resilience and fostering greater well-being in our lives.

Embracing a Breath-Centered Life

In this chapter, we have explored the profound impact that integrating breath into our daily lives can have on our overall well-being. By creating a breath-centered lifestyle, we can navigate life's ups and downs with greater ease and composure. Practicing Breathwork techniques, such as mindful breathing, box breathing, and coherent breathing, helps us manage stress, improve relationships, and build resilience.

Breathwork is particularly valuable in specific situations such as work, relationships, and challenging circumstances. Techniques like 4-4-6 breathing and diaphragmatic breathing can help us stay calm and focused at work, improve communication in our relationships, and provide stability and 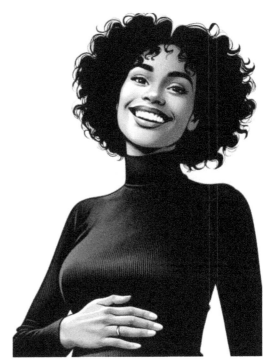 resilience during difficult times.

By cultivating resilience through breath awareness, we develop the inner strength needed to overcome challenges and bounce back from adversity. Remember, the goal is not perfection but finding moments throughout the day to pause, breathe, and reconnect with ourselves. Through consistent practice, we can harness the power of our breath to enhance our overall quality of life.

9
INNER CALM IS A BREATH AWAY

"The greatest weapon against stress is our ability to choose one thought over another."

- William James

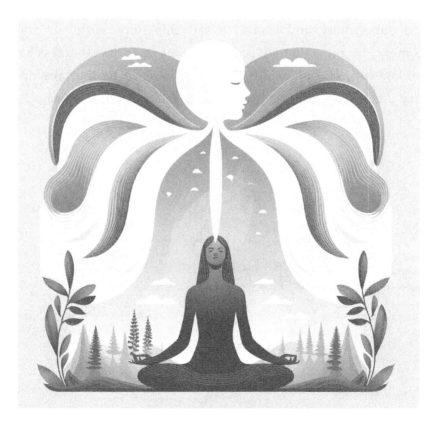

The Power of Every Breath

Although modern life is filled with chronic stress significantly impacting our health, it is evident that the simple act of breathing, something we do every moment without thought, holds profound power. Each breath carries the potential to transform our physical, mental, and emotional well-being. Inner calm is truly just a breath away. By embracing the power of every breath, we can unlock a deeper sense of peace, resilience, and connection to ourselves and the world around us.

In modern times, we're experiencing a stress epidemic which is leading to high rates of chronic conditions that erode our bodies, trauma being passed from generation to generation, and incoherence spreading contagiously between people. We have the opportunity and choice to say 'this stops with me' and commit to preventative self-care using our most accessible remote control: our breath. We can choose to be the presence that lifts a room, calms a friend, and inspires action in others.

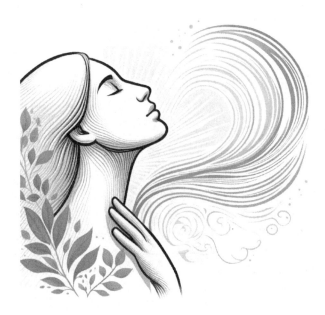

Throughout this book, the intricate connections between breath, stress, and overall well-being have been uncovered. Each chapter has contributed to a holistic understanding of how intentional breathing can transform our lives. From understanding the science behind breath to exploring various techniques and integrating them into daily life, this book can provide a comprehensive toolkit for managing stress and enhancing health.

By fostering a daily practice of breath awareness, we can transform not only our own life but also have a profound impact on our surroundings. Choosing to live with greater intention and mindfulness enables us to cultivate a healthier, more harmonious existence both for ourselves and for those around us.

Breathwork and Self-Discovery: Connecting with Our Inner Wisdom

Breathwork is a powerful tool for self-discovery, helping us connect with our inner wisdom, discernment, and authentic self. Through conscious breathing and inner exploration, we can access deeper layers of consciousness, uncover hidden truths, and cultivate a deeper sense of self-awareness and empowerment. Here's how Breathwork can facilitate self-discovery:

Accessing the Subconscious: Transformational Breathwork can help us access the subconscious mind, where our deepest beliefs, emotions, and memories are stored. By engaging in deep breathing and relaxation techniques, we can bypass the analytical mind and access the deeper layers of our psyche. This can allow us to uncover and process unresolved issues, traumas, and patterns that may be holding us back.

Connecting with Inner Guidance: Breathwork can help us connect to our inner guidance system, which often speaks to us through subtle feelings, sensations, and insights. By quieting the mind and tuning into our breath, we can create space for higher wisdom to emerge. This can help us make decisions, solve problems, and navigate life's challenges with greater clarity and confidence.

Cultivating Self-Awareness: Breathwork fosters self-awareness by bringing our attention to the present moment and our inner experiences. By observing the sensations of our breath and the thoughts and emotions that arise, we can develop a deeper understanding of ourselves and how we relate to the world around us. This self-awareness is essential for personal growth, healing, and transformation as well as combating the chronic stress of modern life.

Releasing Blocks and Limitations: Breathwork can help us release blocks, limitations, and negative patterns that may be hindering our growth and potential. By breathing consciously and with intention, we can create a powerful energetic flow that 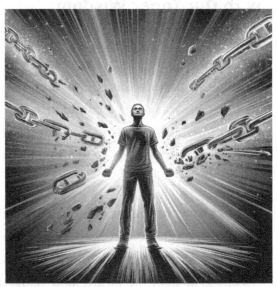 dissolves stuck energy and opens us to new possibilities. This can lead to greater freedom, creativity, and fulfillment in all areas of life.

Embracing Authenticity:

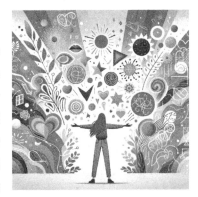

Breathwork invites us to embrace our authenticity and live in alignment with our true selves. By connecting with our breath and inner wisdom, we can clarify our values, desires, and purpose, and align our actions with our highest aspirations. This alignment fosters a sense of wholeness, integrity, and fulfillment, allowing us to live with greater integrity and purpose.

Breathwork is a potent tool for self-discovery, helping us connect with our inner wisdom, higher knowing, and authenticity. By engaging in conscious breathing and inner exploration, we can combat the stressors of life as we access deeper layers of consciousness, release limitations, and cultivate a deeper sense of self-awareness, empowerment, and fulfillment.

Reflecting on the Transformative Power of Breath

Throughout this journey, we've explored the incredible transformative power of breath. From its ability to calm the mind and body to its profound impact on physical, mental, emotional, and even spiritual well-being, breath has shown itself to be a potent tool for inner transformation. We've delved into the science behind Breathwork, explored its practical applications in managing stress and promoting health, and examined its deeper spiritual dimensions. Along the way, we've witnessed how conscious breathing can unlock our innate potential, fostering greater self-awareness, resilience, and vitality.

Committing to a Breath-Centered Life for Personal and Collective Flourishing

As we conclude our exploration, let us commit to embracing a breath-centered life for our personal and collective flourishing. Recognize the power we hold within us—the power to regulate our own nervous system, to cultivate inner calm amidst life's challenges, and to access our innate wisdom and resilience. By prioritizing our breath and integrating Breathwork practices into our daily lives, we can nurture our well-being, enhance our relationships, and contribute to a more compassionate and resilient society.

To keep the concepts discussed in this book active in your daily life, consider the breath not just as a vital life force but as a conscious choice. Understand its power to affect and change your emotional state, offering you the ability to pause and "take a breath" before reacting to any stressful stimulus. Use your new breath remote control to change your emotional state at will.

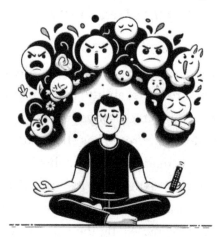

You don't simply have to breathe to live—you have the choice to be aware of your breath and harness its transformative power.

After reading this book, you possess a new knowledge, but the real question is: will you use it? Making the choice to become breath aware is the first step in allowing your breath to change your life for the better. Here are practical ways to incorporate this awareness into your everyday routine:

Start a Breath Journal: Explore the difference between the days when you are mindful of your breath versus the days you are not. Note changes in your happiness and stress levels, your sleep quality, and your reactions to daily challenges.

Set Breath Alarms: Throughout your day, set alarms to pause and check in with your breathing. Use these moments to perform a brief breathing exercise—even 90 seconds can make a significant difference. Track these experiences in your breath journal to notice the subtle impacts on your well-being.

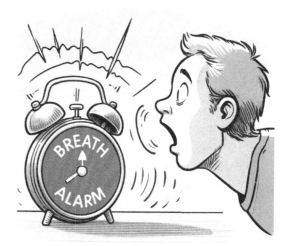

Try out Transformational Breathwork:

Transformational Breathwork is not an everyday practice but can accelerate your path to wellness more quickly than many other healing modalities. Discover more resources at the end of this book and at TheBreathMD.com.

Increase Your CO2 Tolerance: Chronic overbreathing exacerbates stress and anxiety. Developing a practice to increase your CO2 tolerance daily is essential for long-term health and well-being. By changing your dysfunctional breathing patterns, you improve your resilience, mental clarity, and overall physical health. Refer to Chapter 4 and additional information can be found on TheBreathMD.com.

Use Your Breath in Difficult Situations: Prepare for challenging situations with Breathwork. Before entering a stressful environment, take a few minutes to regulate your breathing. This preparation can help you manage stress more effectively and respond with greater calm and clarity. And always remember the power of the pause. Take a moment before responding. Be the calm in the midst of the chaos.

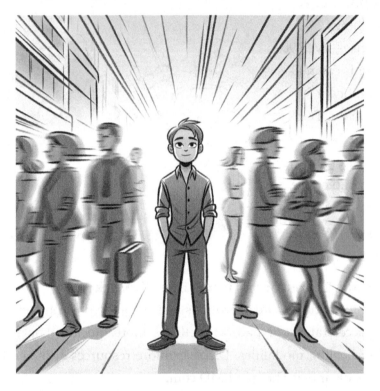

By embracing these practices, you make a decisive choice to use your breath as a tool for personal growth and peace. Let this book be a guide that you take with you, a constant reminder of the power of your breath. Each mindful breath you take is a step toward a life filled with inner calm and well-being. Embrace a breath-centered life and discover how the simple act of breathing can transform not only your own life but also the world around you.

Final thoughts and Encouragement for Your Journey to Inner Calm and Vitality

As we conclude, remember that inner calm is always within reach, accessible through the mindful practice of Breathwork. Embrace the knowledge and techniques shared in this book to help cultivate a state of tranquility and resilience. My journey from "Stressful Chaos to Breath Work Bliss" is a testament to the transformative power of breath.

Take a moment each day to connect with your breath, to be present, and to nurture your inner calm. The path to a more balanced, healthier life begins with a single breath. Breathe deeply, live fully, and discover the peace that lies within.

As you embark on this journey towards inner calm and vitality, know that you are not alone. The path of breath awareness is a deeply personal and transformative journey—one that unfolds in its own time and in its own unique way. As you continue to explore and deepen your relationship with your breath, 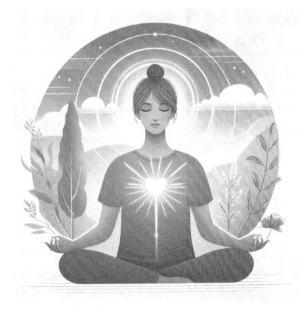 remember to be patient and gentle with yourself. Allow yourself to embrace the process of self-discovery and growth with openness and curiosity. Know that each breath you take is an opportunity to reconnect with yourself, to ground yourself in the present moment, and to tap into your inner resources for strength and resilience. Trust in the wisdom of your breath and the innate intelligence of your body. Allow yourself to surrender to the natural rhythm of your breath, knowing that it holds the key to greater peace, vitality, and well-being.

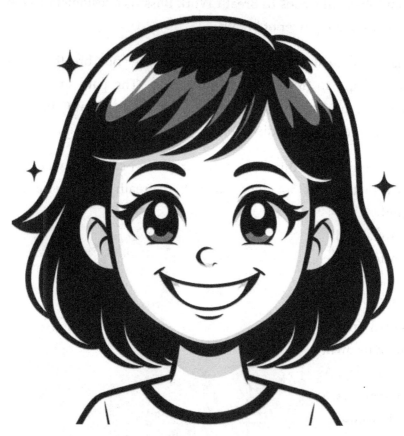

As you navigate life's ups and downs, may you find solace in the steady rhythm of your breath. May you draw upon its calming presence to navigate challenges with grace and ease. And may you cultivate a deep sense of inner calm and vitality that radiates outward, touching the lives of those around you and contributing to the collective well-being of our world.

I invite you to continue exploring and practicing Breathwork. Check out TheBreathMD community to find other like-minded people. Let each breath be a step toward a life filled with inner calm and well-being. Embrace a breath-centered life and find that your inner peace is always just a breath away.

In closing, I offer you these words of encouragement: Trust in the power of your breath. Embrace the journey towards inner calm and vitality with courage and conviction. And know that, with each mindful breath you take, you are stepping into the fullness of your being and aligning yourself with the ever-present flow of life. May your breath be your guide, your anchor, and your source of strength as you continue on your path towards greater well-being and wholeness.

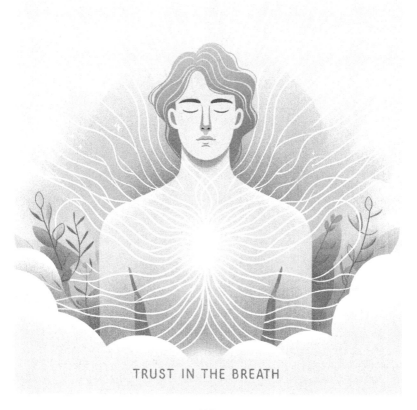

TRUST IN THE BREATH

RESOURCES TO CONTINUE YOUR JOURNEY

"Breath: The New Science of a Lost Art" by James Nestor
- Publisher: Riverhead Books
- Publication Date: May 26, 2020
- ISBN: 978-0735213616
- Description: This book explores the science and history of breathing, offering insights into how modern humans have lost the ability to breathe correctly and how to reclaim this essential skill for better health and well-being. It is a fascinating book, and I highly recommend it.

"The Oxygen Advantage" by Patrick McKeown
- Publisher: William Morrow Paperbacks
- Publication Date: September 15, 2015
- ISBN: 978-0062349477
- Description: Patrick McKeown presents a comprehensive guide on how to improve athletic performance, lose weight, and boost overall health through proper breathing techniques. Breathe Light to Breathe Right.

"The Healing Power of the Breath" by Richard Brown and Patricia Gerbarg

- Publisher: Shambhala
- Publication Date: April 9, 2012
- ISBN: 978-1590309025
- Description: This book provides practical breathing techniques to alleviate stress, anxiety, and depression, supported by scientific research and clinical practice.

"Just Breathe: Mastering Breathwork for Success in Life, Love, Business, and Beyond" by Dan Brulé
- Publisher: TarcherPerigee
- Publication Date: March 28, 2017
- ISBN: 978-1501163064
- Description: Dan Brulé shares techniques and practices to harness the power of breath for personal and professional success.

"Science of Breath: A Practical Guide" by Swami Rama, Rudolph Ballentine, and Alan Hymes

- Publisher: Himalayan Institute Press
- Publication Date: May 25, 1998
- ISBN: 978-0893891510
- Description: This book integrates the science and practice of Breathwork from a yogic perspective, providing practical exercises and insights into the physiological and psychological benefits of breath control.

"The Breath Cure: Develop New Habits for a Healthier, Happier & Longer Life" by Patrick McKeown

- Publisher: Humanix Books
- Publication Date: 2021
- ISBN: 978-1630061975
- Description: Patrick McKeown outlines techniques to develop healthier breathing habits for improved well-being, drawing on decades of scientific research. It has been called "The Breath Bible."

"The Wim Hof Method: Activate Your Full Human Potential" by Wim Hof

- Publisher: Sounds True
- Publication Date: October 20, 2020
- ISBN: 978-1683644095
- Description: Wim Hof shares his method of cold exposure, conscious breathing, and mental focus to unlock human potential and improve health. Educational while entertaining.

"When the Body Says No: The Cost of Hidden Stress" by Gabor Mate, MD

- Publisher: Vintage Canada
- Publication Date: 2003
- ISBN: 978-0676973129
- Description: Dr. Gabor Mate explores the connection between stress and chronic illness, providing insights into the body's response to hidden stress and the devastating results including cancer, dementia, and many others.

"Waking the Tiger: Healing Trauma" by Dr. Peter Levine

- Publisher: North Atlantic Books
- Publication Date: 1997
- ISBN: 978-1556432330
- Description: This book offers a new approach to healing trauma, focusing on the body's natural ability to recover from traumatic experiences. It is widely praised for its groundbreaking approach to trauma therapy through somatic experiencing.

"The Body Keeps the Score: Brain, Mind, and Body in the Healing of Trauma" by Bessel Van Der Kolk, MD

- Publisher: Penguin Books
- Publication Date: 2014
- ISBN: 978-0143127741
- Description: Dr. Bessel Van Der Kolk provides a comprehensive look at how trauma affects the body and mind, and offers new treatments for recovery. It explains the scientific evidence of the mind-body connection and the importance of how trauma affects not only the mind but the body.

"Breathwork: How to Use Your Breath to Change Your Life" by Andrew Smart

- Publisher: Chronicle Books
- Publication Date: 2020
- ISBN: 978-1797200981
- Description: Andrew Smart explores various Breathwork techniques and their benefits for health and well-being.

"Breathe In Breathe Out: Restore Your Health, Reset Your Mind and Find Happiness Through Breathwork" by Stuart Sandeman

- Publisher: Hanover Square Press
- Publication Date: 2022
- ISBN: 978-1335919954
- Description: Stuart Sandeman provides practical Breathwork exercises to improve health, reduce stress, and find happiness.

"The Polyvagal Theory: Neurophysiological Foundations of Emotions, Attachment, Communication, Self-Regulation" by Stephen W. Porges

- Publisher: W. W. Norton & Company
- Publication Date: 2011
- ISBN: 978-0393707007
- Description: Stephen Porges explains The Polyvagal Theory, which describes how the nervous system regulates emotional/physiological states. This is a very dense read written for medical professionals. It was absolutely fascinating but goes into the specifics on a neuroanotomical level so may not be for everyone.

"Body by Breath" by Jill Miller

- Publisher: Victory Belt Publishing Inc.
- Publication Date: 2023
- ISBN: 978-1628604464
- Description: Jill Miller offers a guide to using Breathwork for physical and mental well-being.

"Exhale: 40 Breathwork Exercises to Help You Find Your Calm, Supercharge Your Health, and Perform at Your Best" by Richie Bostock

- Publisher: Penguin Life
- Publication Date: 2020
- ISBN: 978-0241404422
- Description: Richie Bostock provides 40 Breathwork exercises to enhance health and performance.

"Breathing for Warriors" by Dr. Belisa Vranich and Brian Sabin

- Publisher: St. Martin's Essentials
- Publication Date: 2020
- ISBN: 978-1250308224
- Description: This book offers Breathwork techniques specifically designed for athletes and those looking to improve physical performance.

"Holotropic Breathwork: A New Approach to Self-Exploration and Therapy" by Stanislav Grof & Christina Grof
- Publisher: Excelsior Editions
- Publication Date: 2010
- ISBN: 978-1438433992
- Description: Stanislav and Christina Grof introduce holotropic Breathwork, a powerful technique for self-exploration and healing.

"The Illuminated Breath " by Dylan Werner
- Publisher: Victory Belt Publishing
- Publication Date: January 24, 2023
- ISBN: 978-1628605006
- Description: This book teaches you to transform your physical, cognitive, and emotional well-being by harnessing the science of ancient yoga breath practices.

Breathwork Mentors

Brian Kelly
- Role: Co-founder of BreathMasters
- Location: Bali

Steven Jaggers
- Role: Co-founder of Somatiq Breathwork
- Location: Austin, Texas

Witalij Martynow
- Role: Founder of Witality Breathwork
- Location: Los Angeles, California

Niraj Naik
- Role: Founder of Soma Breath
- Location: Lancashire, England

TheBreathMD Services and Packages

Visit www.TheBreathMD.com to learn more.

Free 90-Second Remote Control to Inner Calm – A free video featuring Dr. Jeannie May teaching how to calm your emotional state in just 90 seconds through guided Breathwork.

30 Days to Breathing Free – A series of instructional videos, including follow-along Breathwork sessions with Dr. Jeannie May, designed to teach you multiple cleansing breath techniques for creating a new daily breathing habit for increased energy, emotional regulation, and mental clarity.

Rest and Refresh –A collection of instructional videos and audio recordings designed to ease the symptoms of both types of insomnia: trouble falling asleep and trouble staying asleep. Improve your rest with breath techniques and audio recordings to help you get the sleep you need. If you haven't gotten enough sleep, listen to an audio recording that uses Breathwork and guided meditation to convince your body you've had an extra two hours of restorative sleep, then listen to a short wake-up Breathwork session to energize you for a great day.

Stress Relief –This comprehensive course focuses on increasing CO_2 tolerance for long-term stress relief. It includes a Transformational Breathwork Journey designed for emotional regulation and trauma release, as well as a Restorative Breathwork Journey aimed at achieving balance and peace.

Personalized Breathwork Journey – Experience a recorded, individualized, one-on-one Breathwork Journey with Dr. Jeannie May.

Stay tuned for more to come at TheBreathMD.com!

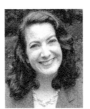

ABOUT THE AUTHOR

Dr. Jeannie May, formerly known as Jean Lessly, M.D., was born and raised in Chattanooga, TN, and currently resides in Nashville. A proud alumnus of The Baylor School, Dr. Jeannie May pursued higher education at Vassar College before earning a medical degree from Washington University School of Medicine. Completing an Internal Medicine Residency and a Geriatric Fellowship at Vanderbilt University, Dr. Jeannie May has obtained board-certifications in Internal Medicine, Geriatrics, Hospice and Palliative Medicine, and Addiction Medicine. She has also become certified in two different types of Breathwork for releasing unprocessed emotions and trapped traumas.

With a passion for adventure, Dr. Jeannie May enjoys hang gliding at Lookout Mountain Flight Park near Chattanooga. As a dedicated parent, Dr. Jeannie May presently has one daughter out of college, two daughters in college, one son in college, and one son in high school.

Dr. Jeannie May turned to writing as a form of therapy after experiencing significant financial and emotional hardship because of embezzlement from her medical practice. Writing under the pseudonym Nicole Kelly, M.D., Dr. Jeannie May has authored two award-winning books that explore the inner workings of sociopaths' minds.

Driven by a mission to make Breathwork a widely recognized and utilized tool for healing, Dr. Jeannie May aims to bridge the wisdom of Western and Ancient Medicine. By promoting the power of breath and fostering community through TheBreathMD, Dr. Jeannie May seeks to empower millions to achieve a holistic sense of well-being in mind, body, and spirit.

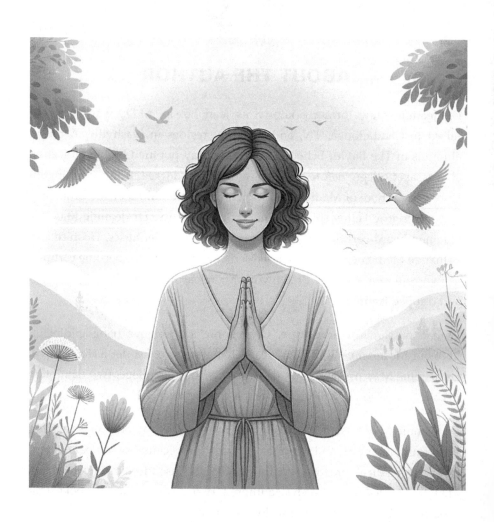

Welcome to TheBreathMD Community

Made in the USA
Middletown, DE
23 August 2024